P9-DUT-348

Headache
and Chronic Pain Syndromes

CURRENT CLINICAL PRACTICE

NEIL S. SKOLNIK, MD SERIES EDITOR

Headache and Chronic Pain Syndromes

The Case-Based Guide to Targeted Assessment and Treatment

Dawn A. Marcus, MD

Pain Institute, University of Pittsburgh
Pittsburgh, PA

HUMANA PRESS ✳ TOTOWA, NEW JERSEY

© 2007 Humana Press Inc.
999 Riverview Drive, Suite 208
Totowa, New Jersey 07512

humanapress.com

All rights reserved. No part of this book may be reproduced, stored in a retrieval system, or transmitted in any form or by any means, electronic, mechanical, photocopying, microfilming, recording, or otherwise without written permission from the Publisher.

All papers, comments, opinions, conclusions, or recommendations are those of the author(s), and do not necessarily reflect the views of the publisher.

Due diligence has been taken by the publishers, editors, and authors of this book to assure the accuracy of the information published and to describe generally accepted practices. The contributors herein have carefully checked to ensure that the drug selections and dosages set forth in this text are accurate and in accord with the standards accepted at the time of publication. Notwithstanding, as new research, changes in government regulations, and knowledge from clinical experience relating to drug therapy and drug reactions constantly occurs, the reader is advised to check the product information provided by the manufacturer of each drug for any change in dosages or for additional warnings and contraindications. This is of utmost importance when the recommended drug herein is a new or infrequently used drug. It is the responsibility of the treating physician to determine dosages and treatment strategies for individual patients. Further it is the responsibility of the health care provider to ascertain the Food and Drug Administration status of each drug or device used in their clinical practice. The publisher, editors, and authors are not responsible for errors or omissions or for any consequences from the application of the information presented in this book and make no warranty, express or implied, with respect to the contents in this publication.

This publication is printed on acid-free paper. ∞
ANSI Z39.48-1984 (American Standards Institute) Permanence of Paper for Printed Library Materials.

Production Editor: Robin B. Weisberg

Cover design by Patricia F. Cleary

For additional copies, pricing for bulk purchases, and/or information about other Humana titles, contact Humana at the above address or at any of the following numbers: Tel.: 973-256-1699; Fax: 973-256-8341; E-mail: orders@humanapr.com; or visit our Website: www.humanapress.com

Photocopy Authorization Policy:

Photocopy Authorization Policy: Authorization to photocopy items for internal or personal use, or the internal or personal use of specific clients is granted by Humana Press, provided that the base fee of US $30.00 per copy is paid directly to the Copyright Clearance Center (CCC), 222 Rosewood Dr., Danvers MA 01923. For those organizations that have been granted a photocopy license from the CCC, a separate system of payment has been arranged and is acceptable to the Humana Press. The fee code for users of the Transactional Reporting Service is 1-58829-745-4/07 $30.00.

Printed in the United States of America. 10 9 8 7 6 5 4 3 2 1

eISBN 1-59745-258-0

Library of Congress Cataloging-in-Publication Data

Marcus, Dawn A.
  Headache and chronic pain syndromes : the case-based guide to targeted assessment and treatment / Dawn A. Marcus.
     p. ; cm. -- (Current clinical practice)
  Includes bibliographical references and index.
  ISBN 1-58829-745-4 (alk. paper)
  1. Headache--Case studies. 2. Chronic pain--Case studies.
  [DNLM: 1. Chronic Disease--Case Reports. 2. Pain--etiology--Case Reports.
3. Headache--therapy--Case Reports. 4. Pain--therapy--Case Reports. WL 704 M322h 2007]
I. Title. II. Series.
  RC392.M37 2006
  616'.0472--dc22
                                                                    2006004457

Series Editor's Introduction

As physicians and clinicians, we are all well aware that Congress declared the years 2000 through 2010 as the Decade of Pain Control and Research. From a primary care standpoint, pain in one form or another is the chief complaint of most of the patients we see. Accordingly, it is critical for us to keep abreast of best practices in diagnosing and treating painful syndromes. Chronic pain is a special problem. Pain signals keep firing in the nervous system for weeks, months, even years. There may have been an initial injury—sprained back, serious infection—or there may be an ongoing cause of pain such as arthritis, cancer, or ear infection. In addition, making matters more complicated, some people suffer chronic pain in the absence of any past injury or evidence of body damage. All of this makes chronic pain syndromes perhaps our most problematic clinical cases.

Headache and Chronic Pain Syndromes: The Case-Based Guide to Targeted Assessment and Treatment by Dr. Dawn Marcus seeks to improve this situation. This concise title provides the primary care physician and clinicians with a clear, organized approach to the evaluation and management of chronic pain. Importantly, Dr. Marcus discusses pain management from the point of view of the busy clinician, using a case-based approach to make the information relevant and memorable. In this book it is evident that Dr. Marcus clearly understands the challenges that are faced by both patients and the physicians who care for them, and presents us with a much-needed, organized way to approach this common and difficult problem. For that, the medical community should be most grateful. I am pleased to welcome this resource into the *Current Clinical Practice* series.

Neil S. Skolnik, MD
Associate Director
Family Practice Residency Program
Abington Memorial Hospital
Abington, PA
Professor of Family and Community Medicine
Temple University School of Medicine
Philadelphia, PA

Preface

When I looked at the charts for my first three patients this morning, everyone looked the same—several weeks of neck pain and x-rays diagnosing degenerative disease. I've got to be able to quickly sort through each patient. All I can tell from their charts is that each one's a pain in the neck.

In medical school, we learned to obtain a chief complaint and an undirected history, allowing the patient to provide information about his or her condition without using excessive focused questions. Although this approach prevents the examiner from concentrating on an incorrect diagnosis before enough facts have been identified, it is time-consuming and fails to direct the patient to important historical information. In addition, an unfocused evaluation often identifies nonspecific or unrelated abnormalities.

In a busy clinic, accurate diagnoses are generally reached by using the chief complaint to select an appropriate targeted history and physical examination. This targeted approach helps gather information to distinguish among common conditions that result in the chief complaint. The same general elements are used in the target examination for all chronic pain complaints, although the details vary based on pain location. Targeting the evaluation avoids excessive cost and wasted time associated with testing not directed toward specific diagnoses.

Headache and Chronic Pain Syndromes: The Case-Based Guide to Targeted Assessment and Treatment is designed to provide targeted assessments and treatment plans for common, chronically painful conditions. These assessments will be applied to typical case scenarios for each area of chronic pain. Using this approach should facilitate expeditious evaluation of pain complaints and the delivery of effective pain treatment.

Dawn A. Marcus, MD

Acknowledgment

I developed the popular feature, "Monday Morning Patients," in the journal *Headache & Pain* in order to highlight the targeted assessment of headache and chronic pain patients. This book uses a similar case-based approach to develop practical and efficient tools for diagnosing and treating chronic pain conditions. I would like to thank Dr. Seymour Diamond for his continued support and efforts to educate clinicians to more effectively manage patients with headache and other chronic pain syndromes.

Please feel free to visit my website, www.dawnmarcusmd.com, for more information and to share any feedback you have on this book.

Contents

Introduction

CHAPTER HIGHLIGHTS

- On average, two of every five patients coming in for a primary care visit have a pain complaint.
- Analgesics and arthritis medications are among the top five medications prescribed to primary care patients.
- Pain becomes chronic (lasting >3 months) in 30% of patients.
- Changes in neural activation and connections result in chronic pain.
- Evaluation and management of chronic pain is most efficient when using a targeted assessment and treatment approach.

* * *

Pain is one of the most common complaints at primary care visits. In a survey of 5646 primary care outpatient visits, pain was listed as a complaint for 40% of patients (Fig. 1; ref. *1*). In this survey, pain interfered with work for 25% of patients and home activities for 13%. Another study of primary care practices in 14 countries recorded interviews for nearly 26,000 consecutive patients *(2)*. In this study, persistent pain was defined as pain that occurred most of the time for at least 6 months. In addition, pain had to be severe enough that the patients sought medical evaluation or treatment, or experienced pain-related disability. In this survey, significant, persistent pain was identified in 25% of women and 16% of men. The most commonly reported pain locations were the back, head, and joints.

Given the high prevalence of pain, it is not surprising that primary care doctors frequently prescribe pain treatments. Data from the 1999 and 2000 National Ambulatory Medical Care Surveys and National Hospital Ambulatory Medical Care Surveys identified anti-arthritics, non-opioid analgesics, and opioid analgesics as three of the top five medication categories prescribed to ambulatory care patients *(3)*. (Antidepressants and vaccines were the other top prescribed medications.) Pain-relieving medication was prescribed or administered for nearly 206 million visits—almost 14% of all ambulatory care visits.

From: *Current Clinical Practice: Headache and Chronic Pain Syndromes: The Case-Based Guide to Targeted Assessment and Treatment*
By: D. A. Marcus © Humana Press, Totowa, NJ

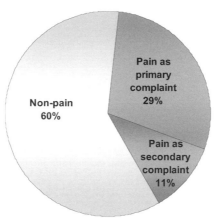

Fig. 1. Percentage of primary care practitioner visits for pain. (Based on ref. 5.)

Despite the high number of pain complaints reported in the typical primary care practice, a recent survey of 161 primary care practitioners showed that only 15% endorsed the statement, "I enjoy working with patients who have chronic nonmalignant pain" *(4)*. Lack of comfort and enthusiasm for managing patients with chronic pain may be related to the following perceptions:

• Pain evaluations are time-consuming.
• Assignment of chronic pain diagnoses is arbitrary.
• Pain treatments are ineffective.
• Patients reporting chronic pain are looking for drugs of abuse.

Increased understanding about the physiology, evaluation, and treatment of chronic pain should help dispel these myths and improve physician comfort with treating patients suffering from pain.

1. DISTINGUISHING ACUTE FROM CHRONIC PAIN

Acute pain is a common sequela of injury or illness. Acute pain generally lessens shortly after onset, and is completely gone when healing is complete (Fig. 2). Chronic pain, however, persists for more than 3 months. This is the pain that lasts beyond the time of healing after an acute illness or injury. Chronic pain may also occur in patients with ongoing degenerative illnesses, such as rheumatoid arthritis, or other chronic conditions, such as migraine. Pain severity may fluctuate in patients with chronic pain, with times of increased pain or pain flares occurring either in relation to increased activity or stress, or insidiously. As described here, chronic pain occurs as a result of persistent activation of neural pain pathways and muscle spasms.

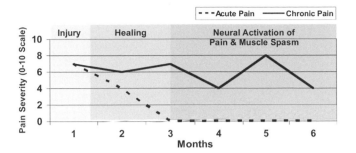

Fig. 2. Acute versus chronic pain. Acute pain occurs with trauma or illness, generally decreasing during the period of healing. Acute pain usually resolves within 3 months. Chronic pain persists after healing is completed owing to continued activation of neural pain pathways and muscle spasm.

Although most pain complaints will resolve within 3 months, a survey of patients seeing their primary care practitioners for pain showed pain lasting more than 3 months in 30% of patients and more than 6 months in 21% of patients (Fig. 3; ref. 5). Pain was experienced frequently in most patients, with daily chronic pain occurring in 20% of patients.

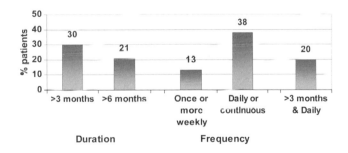

Fig. 3. Pain characteristics in primary care patients. (Based on ref. 5.)

2. UNDERSTANDING THE PHYSIOLOGY OF CHRONIC PAIN

The persistence of pain complaints long after an injury, successful surgery, or healing leads to skepticism about the veracity of patients' pain reports. Even when health care providers believe their patients have pain, they often feel that patients are exaggerating their complaints. An interesting study compared pain scores assigned by patients and their general practitioners, using a 5-point severity scale *(5)*. Doctors rated their patients' pain intensity at least one level

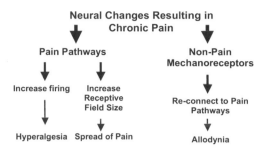

Fig. 4. Pathophysiology of chronic pain. Exposure to acute pain, in some cases, results in activation of neural pathways that persist long-term. Increased firing of pain pathways results in increased pain severity (hyperalgesia). Enlargement of neural receptive fields results in the spread of pain to contiguous, previously unaffected body areas. Mechanoreceptors disconnect from tactile pathways and connect to pain pathways. This results in nonpainful touch stimuli being perceived as pain (allodynia).

lower than the patients did at 37% of the patient visits, and two levels lower at 20% of visits.

Experimental studies now confirm that changes in neural activity and neural connections are responsible for persistent pain that lasts beyond the period of healing. Exposing a laboratory rat to a temporary nerve injury by tying a ligature around a nerve in an extremity and then removing it results in no loss of sensory or motor function. The rat, however, will display chronic pain behaviors by biting its limb *(6,7)*. When these rats are examined physiologically and micro-scopically, a variety of changes in neural activity and morphology are identified that result in persistent pain (Fig. 4; refs. *8* and *9*). Activity from free nerve endings is heightened, resulting in a lower pain threshold and greater pain response, or *hyperalgesia*. Enlargement of neuronal receptive fields produces hyperalgesia in uninjured areas adjacent to the areas served by the affected nerve. In addition, mechanoreceptor neurons that respond to nonpainful tactile stimuli in the normal rat rewire to connect with pain pathways. This results in activation of pain pathways and *allodynia*, the cerebral perception of pain after exposure to light touch or vibration.

Although these pain experiments have not been reproduced in humans, many of the pain responses seen in humans with chronic pain are strikingly similar to those in the laboratory rat. For example, these same neural changes may explain the persistent pain (hyperalgesia) after successful removal of a herniated disc in a patient with neck or back pain. Patients may also report that their pain initially only affected their ankle, but months later the whole foot is bothering them (spread of pain to noninjured areas). Finally, patients with neuropathic pain typically describe pain resulting from the bedclothes brushing their limb or the examiner's gentlest touch (allodynia).

Why chronic pain occurs only in some people and not in others with similar injuries or health problems has not been explained. These animal experiments, however, do help to confirm the legitimacy of patients' pain complaints, even after successful surgery or healing when laboratory and radiographic studies may be normal.

3. DEVELOPING A TARGETED ASSESSMENT

Evaluating patients with complicated chronic pain is facilitated by using a highly focused, targeted approach. A targeted assessment should focus on high-yield questions and examination findings to help distinguish among common causes of chronic pain. Although it may seem quicker to "just scan everything," many tests become "abnormal" with the normal aging process and result in further costly and time-consuming evaluations, tests, and consultations. For example, although a magnetic resonance imaging (MRI) scan of the brain will reassure a patient with a migraine that he or she does not have a brain tumor, about 30% of migraine sufferers will have nonspecific white matter abnormalities on MRI scan that raise questions about the need for additional testing for multiple sclerosis, strokes, and tumors *(10)*. Similarly, radiographic abnormalities of the spine are often not clinically significant. For example, MRI scans in asymptomatic adults in their 20s show disc degeneration in 29% in the cervical spine and 34% in the lumbar spine *(11,12)*. Bulging discs are seen in 32% in the cervical spine and 6% in the lumbar spine. Abnormal MRI scans become more prevalent in asymptomatic controls with increased age. Interestingly, disc protrusion or herniation is not necessarily related to the likelihood of back pain in younger or older adults *(12)*. Likewise, abnormalities are also frequently identified in asymptomatic controls imaged with computed tomography (CT). In a group of 52 controls, 35% had abnormal lumbar studies, with the percentage of abnormalities increasing to 50% after the age of 40 years *(13)*. In controls younger than 40 years of age, 20% had CT scans that revealed herniated discs.

Although a unique targeted assessment will be provided in this book for every pain location, similar principles apply to these assessments (Table 1). The targeted assessment is helpful to expedite identifying a diagnosis and to avoid obtaining unnecessary tests that may reveal nonspecific abnormalities that may confuse the diagnosis.

After identifying pain as a chief complaint, all patients should complete a pain drawing (Fig. 5). Patients should be asked to note *all* of their pain complaints, not only those that are the most bothersome or that brought them to the clinic. For example, the diagnosis and treatment will be very different for

Table 1
Developing a Targeted Pain Assessment

• History	○ Clarify the pain location: complete a pain drawing
	○ Identify precipitants to the pain
	○ Identify additional medical conditions
	○ Complete a review of systems
• Physical examination	○ Neurological examination focusing on gait and extremity strength, reflexes, and sensation
	○ Musculoskeletal examination looking for areas of tenderness and assessing joint mobility
	○ General medical examination as appropriate
• Laboratory and radiological testing	○ Possible blood work for systemic illness or inflammatory disease
	○ Possible X-rays for bony abnormalities
	○ Possible MRIs for neurological disorders
	○ Possible EMG/NCV for peripheral nerve disease

MRI, magnetic resonance imaging; EMG, electromyography; NCV, nerve conduction velocity.

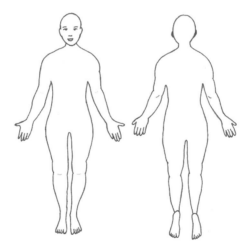

Fig. 5. Pain drawing recording sheet. Patients are instructed to shade all painful areas, using the following key: //// = pain; :::::: = numbness; **** = burning or hypersensitivity (Reprinted with permission from ref. *14*.)

two 35-year-old women who come to the office with a chief complaint of migraine (Fig. 6). Although both describe typical migraine headaches, one has migraine with fibromyalgia, which will require more comprehensive treatment than the other woman who has isolated migraine.

After likely disorders that commonly cause pain are identified, targeted testing can be performed to rule in or out specific disorders. General screening

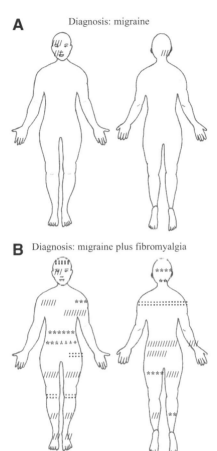

Fig. 6. Pain drawings in two women with the chief complaint of migraine. (**A**) Diagnosis: migraine. (**B**) Diagnosis: migraine plus fibromyalgia.

tests for chronic pain are expensive and frequently reveal insignificant or nonspecific abnormalities that are unrelated to the chronic pain condition.

4. TARGETED CHRONIC PAIN MANAGEMENT

Pain management can be divided into treatments designed to alleviate or minimize long-term pain complaints (restorative treatments), treatment to prevent future occurrences/recurrences of pain (preventive therapies), and thera-

Table 2
Developing a Targeted Treatment Plan

	Nonmedication	Medication
• Restorative treatment	Targeted physical therapy	Disease-specific drugs
• Preventive therapies	Relaxation and biofeedback	Disease-specific drugs
	Stress management	Antidepressants
	Cognitive restructuring	Anti-epileptics
	Reconditioning exercises	
	Stretching exercises	
	Pacing skills	
	Body mechanics	
• Flare techniques	Relaxation techniques	Disease-specific drugs
	Trigger-point compression	Non-opioid analgesics
	Stretching exercises	Opioid analgesics

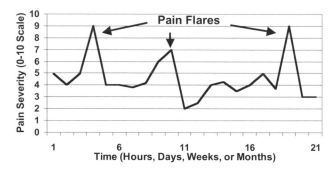

Fig. 7. Typical pattern of chronic pain.

pies to treat severe increases in pain severity (flare techniques; *see* Table 2). Within each treatment category, effective medication and nonmedication treatments may be utilized.

Treatment outcome can be readily assessed by comparing pre- and post-treatment pain drawings and pain severity scores. An 11-point pain severity score (0 = *no pain*, 10 = *excruciating*) is readily understood by patients and correlates with global improvement assessments *(15)*. A reduction in pain of at least 2 points on this scale denotes significant improvement, rated by patients as much or very much improved. Mapping pain severity scores can help recognize typical daily pain severity, as well as frequency and duration of pain flares (Fig. 7).

In this book, each chapter will cover disease-specific treatments. General chronic pain management techniques are described in Chapter 11, along with patient educational materials. Typically, both disease-specific and general chronic pain treatments are used for most chronically painful conditions.

REFERENCES

1. Mäntyselkä P, Kumpusalo E, Ahonen R, et al. Pain as a reason to visit the doctor: a study in Finnish primary health care. Pain 2001;89:175–180.
2. Gureje O, Von Korff M, Simon GE, Gater R. Persistent pain and well-being. A World Health Organization study in primary care. JAMA 1998;280:147–151.
3. Burt CW, Schappert SM. Ambulatory care visits to physician offices, hospital outpatient departments, and emergency departments: United States, 1999–2000. Vital Health Stat 13 2004;157:1–70.
4. Potter M, Schafer S, Gonzalez-Mendez E, et al. Opioids for chronic nonmalignant pain: attitudes and practices of primary care physicians in the UCSFG/Stanford Collaborative Research Network. J Fam Pract 2001;50:145–151.
5. Mäntyselkä P, Kumpusalo E, Ahonen R, Takala J. Patients' versus general practitioners' assessments of pain intensity in primary care patients with non-cancer pain. Br J Gen Pract 2001;51:995–997.
6. Bennett GJ, Xie YK. A peripheral mononeuropathy in rat that produces disorders of pain sensation like those seen in man. Pain 1988;33:87–107.
7. Seltzer Z, Dubner R, Shir Y. A novel behavioral model of neuropathic pain disorders produced in rats by partial sciatic nerve injury. Pain 1990;43:205–218.
8. Guilbaud G, Gautron M, Jazat F, et al. Time course of degeneration and regeneration of myelinated nerve fibers following chronic loose ligatures of the rat sciatic nerve: can nerve lesions be linked to the abnormal pain-related behaviours? Pain 1993;53:147–158.
9. Behbehani MM, Dollberg-Stolik O. Partial sciatic nerve ligation results in an enlargement of the receptive field and enhancement of the response of dorsal horn neurons to noxious stimulation by an adenosine agonist. Pain 1994;58:421–428.
10. Marcus DA. Central nervous system abnormalities in migraine. Expert Opin Pharmacother 2003;4:1709–1715.
11. Siivola SM, Levoska S, Ilkko E, Vanharanta H, Keinänen-Kiukaanniemi S. MRI changes of cervical spine in asymptomatic and symptomatic young adults. Eur Spine J 2002;11:358–363.
12. Savage RA, Whitehouse GH, Roberts N. The relationship between the magnetic resonance imaging appearance of the lumbar spine and low back pain, age and occupation in males. Eur Spine J 1997;6:106–114.
13. Wiesel SW, Tsourmas N, Feffer HL, Citrin CM, Patronas N. A study of computer-assisted tomography. I. The incidence of positive CAT scans in an asymptomatic group of patients. Spine 1984;9:549–551.
14. Marcus DA. Chronic Pain: A Primary Guide to Practical Management. Totowa, NJ: Humana Press, 2005.
15. Farrar JT, Young JP, LaMoreaux L, Werth JL, Poole RM. Clinical importance of changes in chronic pain intensity measured on an 11-point numerical pain rating scale. Pain 2001;94:149–158.

2

Pain in the Head

CHAPTER HIGHLIGHTS

- Key features used to differentiate among common causes of headache include identification of unilateral or bilateral pain, pain duration, and preferred activity or behaviors during a headache episode.
- New-onset headache, headache beginning after age 50, posterior head pain, and neurological complaints each suggest that a work-up for secondary causes of headache will be needed.
- Migraine is the most common chronic headache seen in primary care practices.
- Daily headache diaries are important tools for accurately assessing headache patterns.

* * *

This afternoon, you have five new patients who range in age from 12 to 75 years old. Each patient comes to the office with a chief complaint of *a pain in the head*. They have each diagnosed themselves with sinus headache and have had variable success with over-the-counter (OTC) sinus remedies. They each come to the office seeking antibiotics. Here are the stories each patient tells your nurse:

Patient 1: Mrs. Franklin is a 48-year-old accountant. "I used to get terrible migraines with my menstrual periods. I'd throw up and spend the day in bed with a washcloth over my eyes. My migraines got better after I had my kids, but since I'm starting menopause, I've been getting terrible sinus headaches."

Patient 2: Steven is a 12-year-old seventh-grade student. His mom brought him in for headaches. "Steven only gets headaches during the school year. I'm sure it's just stress and struggling with school. He missed school twice this month already for the headaches, but then he was fine by mid-morning. His headaches are nothing like my migraines, so I'm guessing they're stress or maybe sinus headaches."

From: *Current Clinical Practice: Headache and Chronic Pain Syndromes:*
The Case-Based Guide to Targeted Assessment and Treatment
By: D. A. Marcus © Humana Press, Totowa, NJ

Patient 3: Mr. Hillman is a 45-year-old jazz pianist. "My wife's beginning to think I'm just crazy. These horrid headaches make me want to blow my head off. I only get them in the spring and fall, so my wife thinks they might be allergies from my sinuses. I don't know what I'd do if I got one of these while performing."

Patient 4: Ms. Inglis is a 35-year-old homemaker. "I've had migraines since I was 13, but now I wake up everyday with a headache. They seem to worsen when the weather changes or is about to change, so it's got to be sinuses."

Patient 5: Mrs. Jeffries is a 75-year-old hospital volunteer. "I suffered with migraines my whole life, spending a couple of days every month in bed. These thankfully stopped when I was in my 50s. I can't believe I've started having headaches again. My migraines were like a spike through my eye and these are on my right forehead, so I think my sinuses must be acting up."

1. EVALUATING HEAD PAIN

Although more people in the general population experience a tension-type headache than a migraine, the vast majority of people suffering from headaches seeking treatment actually have migraines. More than 90% of 1203 patients consulting their primary care doctors for headache were diagnosed with migraine as the cause for their complaint *(1)*. Despite the overwhelming prevalence of migraines in primary care patients with a headache, patients themselves are often convinced that their headaches are related to sinus disease. Headache features that are characteristically linked to the sinuses commonly occur in migraine. A clinical assessment of nearly 3000 patients who were self- or physician-diagnosed with sinus headache resulted in a migraine diagnosis in 80% *(2)*. In addition to typical migraine features (such as throbbing pain, photophobia, phonophobia, and nausea), those patients with migraine also endorsed a variety of "sinus" symptoms: sinus pressure (84%), sinus pain (82%), nasal congestion (63%), runny nose (40%), and watery eyes (38%). Moreover, migraine pain usually affects those areas near the facial sinuses. A survey of 1283 migraine patients found the most common pain locations were around the eyes (67%), temple (58%), and forehead (56% *[3]*). About half of migraineurs identify changes in weather as a possible migraine trigger, although only 24% feel that weather changes will *usually* trigger a migraine *(4)*. Interestingly, patients with a migraine with eye pain are more likely to report weather changes as a trigger *(3)*.

Although the chief complaints and brief histories in the five patients mentioned earlier are typical, none has provided enough information to formulate an educated diagnosis. Despite the fact that each patient has the same primary

Table 1
Common Causes of Head Pain

Disease category	Specific diseases
• Idiopathic	○ Migraine ○ Tension-type headache ○ Cluster headache
• Musculoskeletal	○ Temporomandibular dysfunction ○ Cervical myofascial or joint dysfunction
• Inflammatory/ autoimmune	○ Acute infection (e.g., upper respiratory infection, meningitis) ○ Temporal/giant-cell arteritis ○ Systemic lupus erythematosus
• Systemic illness	○ Anemia ○ Thyroid disease
• Intracranial pathology	○ Tumor ○ Vascular malformation or aneurysm ○ Subdural hematoma ○ Cerebrovascular disease

complaint, differences in history and examination can provide ready clues to diagnostic possibilities (Table 1). Although migraine is a very common cause of chronic headache, headaches may be caused by a wide variety of medical conditions. The most common cause of acute or new-onset headache is acute viral or bacterial infection. Trauma is another common cause of new headache. A review of 288 randomly selected cases of children coming to the emergency room with the main complaint of headache showed that headache was caused by upper respiratory tract infections in more than 60% of cases, with migraine accounting for only 16% of headache conditions *(5)*. A similar survey of 150 children visiting an emergency room for severe, acute headache identified a diagnosis of upper respiratory infection in 57% and migraine in only 18% of cases *(6)*. Headache may also occur with viral illnesses and other infections in adults. In older adults, other important causes of acute headache include trauma, hemorrhage, tumor, and giant-cell arteritis. Headache features that suggest intracranial pathology include recent change in headache pattern, patient age over 50 years old, posterior head pain, and additional neurological complaints *(7)*. Extracting important features to distinguish among common disorders depends on a targeted evaluation that focuses on high-yield questions and examination findings that help distinguish among the many possible causes of head pain (Table 2).

Table 2
Distinguishing Characteristics of Common Recurring Headaches

	Location	Duration (hours)	Activity during headache
• Migraine (adults)	Unilateral (affected side should at least occasionally vary)	8–24	Reduced productivity, lays down, seeks dark and quiet retreat
• Migraine (kids)	Bilateral forehead	1–4	Brief curtailment of activity
• Tension-type	Bilateral	8–24 or constant	No interference
• Medication overuse	Bilateral	Constant with fluctuating severity	No interference
• Cluster	Unilateral eye (affected side will never vary)	0.5–1.5	Avoids laying down, paces, smokes, showers, hits head

Table 3
Keys to a Targeted Evaluation of Head Pain

- **History**
  - Clarify pain location—complete pain drawing
  - Clarify duration of headache—new onset versus chronic
  - Note typical activity during headache episode
  - Record pain precipitants
  - Identify pain pattern—intermittent versus constant, duration of each headache episode
  - Identify additional medical conditions
  - Record headache and pain medication usage, including over-the-counter medications
  - Obtain complete review of systems
- **Physical examination**
  - Musculoskeletal exam: ROM and tenderness cervical spine and temporomandibular area
  - Neurological exam: mental status exam, cranial nerve screen (including fundoscopic exam), extremity strength, reflexes, sensation, and gait
- **Testing**
  - Blood tests for medical conditions as indicated (e.g., thyroid tests, autoimmune testing)
  - X-ray of the cervical spine for mechanical signs
  - CT scan or MRI of brain for new-onset worrisome headache or patient with neurological deficits
  - Lumbar puncture if suspicious of bleed or infection
  - Erythrocyte sedimentation rate and temporal artery biopsy in patients with new headache after age 50 without obvious diagnosis

ROM, range of motion; CT, computed tomography; MRI, magnetic resonance imaging.

1.1. Developing a High-Yield Targeted Evaluation of Head Pain

Evaluations of patients with head pain should be targeted to specific likely clinical scenarios to help confirm or refute clinical diagnoses. The same evaluation principles apply to each patient regarding features in the history, physical examination findings, and the need to proceed with testing. Details of the targeted examination are outlined in Table 3. In most cases of chronic headache, pain is focused at the forehead, eyes, and cheeks. Therefore, the pain drawing in patients with a headache is most useful for identifying associated pain conditions, such as fibromyalgia. When the history seems complicated or confusing, ask your patients suffering from headaches to complete daily headache diaries by recording pain severity and medication use for several weeks (Fig. 1). Diaries can help identify headache patterns and triggers. Premonitory changes or prodromes occur in about one-third of migraineurs, typically within 6 hours of headache onset *(8)*. The most common prodromes are fatigue, mood changes, and gastrointestinal symptoms, each occurring in about one-quarter of all migraineurs. Identifying consistent prodromal symptoms allows patients to identify the very early stages of migraine and receive treatment before pain and other disabling symptoms begin.

1.2. Applying the Targeted Exam to Each Patient

Pain drawings showed head pain only in three patients, with additional unrelated low back pain for Ms. Inglis and knee pain for Mrs. Jeffries. The results of the targeted evaluation are provided for each patient in Tables 4–8. Review each patient's findings, decide if additional testing is necessary, and formulate a likely diagnosis. Then read the following sections to compare your interpretations with the patients' diagnoses in the clinic.

1.2.1. Patient 1: Mrs. Franklin—48-Year-Old Accountant (Table 4)

Mrs. Franklin reports intermittent, unilateral headache that changes sides and is associated with reduced work productivity. She retreats to dark, quiet isolation during headache episodes. She also has evidence of cervical musculoskeletal abnormalities, with no neurological deficits. No additional testing was ordered, and she was diagnosed with migraine.

Like Mrs. Franklin, patients often fail to recognize their headaches as migraines, especially if they do not go to bed or vomit with their headaches. The frequent location of migraine and other chronic benign headaches over the sinuses often leads to a misinterpretation of an idiopathic headache disorder as recurring sinusitis or "sinus" headache. In addition, many OTC sinus remedies are also effective for migraine. Most sinus remedies contain an analgesic and an antihistamine. A recent study compared the efficacy of the intravenous, migraine-specific, acute care medication dihydroergotamine (DHE-45) with intravenous diphenhydramine (Benadryl®) in 80 migraineurs *(9)*.

Daily Headache Diary

Name: _____

Date: _____ / _____ / _____

Time of Day	Severity						Medications
	0	1	2	3	4	5	
Morning							
Noon							
Evening							
Bedtime							
List non-medication treatment strategies used:							

Migraine Symptoms
- ❑ One-sided pain
- ❑ Throbbing or pulsing
- ❑ Decreased activities
- ❑ Reduced lights
- ❑ Reduced noises
- ❑ Avoided smells
- ❑ Nauseated or vomited

Prodrome & aura
- ❑ Fatigue
- ❑ Mood change
- ❑ Digestive/stomach problem
- ❑ Neck or head pain
- ❑ Eye problem or vision change
- ❑ Sensitivity to lights or noise
- ❑ Dizziness
- ❑ Difficulty concentrating
- ❑ Food craving
- ❑ Aura
- ❑ _____
- ❑ _____
- ❑ _____

Triggers
- ❑ Menses
- ❑ Stress
- ❑ Glare
- ❑ Skipped a meal
- ❑ Overslept
- ❑ Too little sleep
- ❑ Odor
- ❑ Change in weather
- ❑ Exercise
- ❑ Alcohol
- ❑ Over 2 cups of caffeine beverage
- ❑ Chocolate
- ❑ Tomato/tomato sauce
- ❑ Peanut butter
- ❑ Processed meats
- ❑ Canned food
- ❑ Chinese food
- ❑ Aspartame
- ❑ Broad beans
- ❑ _____
- ❑ _____
- ❑ _____

Fig. 1. Daily headache diary. (Reproduced with permission from ref. *9a*.)

Both treatments effectively reduced migraine pain. Interestingly, diphenhydramine provided better immediate, short-term pain reduction, whereas DHE-45 provided a better accumulated, long-term response.

Musculoskeletal abnormalities frequently occur in patients with migraine, as well as tension-type headache. A comparison of patients with headache and headache-free controls found cervical posture abnormalities in 90% of headache sufferers versus 46% of controls, and myofascial dysfunction in 81% of patients with headaches versus 54% of controls *(10)*. Abnormalities in headache sufferers were similar for patients diagnosed with migraine, tension-type,

Table 4
Results of Targeted Evaluation for Patient 1:
Mrs. Franklin—48-Year-Old Accountant

Targeted assessment	Findings
History	○ Pain usually affects her forehead, eye, and cheek on one side of the head. Pain is usually on the left but occasionally on the right. Sometimes the pain switches sides during an attack.
	○ Headaches began around 13 years old. Headache pattern has been stable for the last 2 years.
	○ Work productivity suffers during a headache. Goes into office and tries to dim lights and be left alone.
	○ Headaches first began with menarche, improved during pregnancy, then worsened when she began getting hot flashes.
	○ Headache is intermittent but occurs about 3 days per week. Each episode lasts about 12 hours.
	○ General health is good.
	○ Over-the-counter sinus remedies are effective if she catches her headache early.
	○ ROS remarkable for obesity.
Physical exam	
• Musculoskeletal	○ Mildly decreased cervical ROM. Bilateral neck tenderness to palpation. Jaw opens without discomfort; masticatory muscles nontender.
• Neurological	○ Normal neurological examination.

ROM, range of motion; ROS, review of systems.

or combined migraine and tension-type headache. Identification of musculoskeletal dysfunction is usually most significantly related to headache pathology for those patients in whom neck motion or palpation directly aggravates or precipitates head pain.

Headache pattern and severity generally change during a patient's lifetime. In women, headaches typically begin with menses, improve with pregnancy, worsen in early menopause, and improve in later menopause *(11)*. Estrogen acts as an important neuromodulator, with cycling affecting several neurotransmitters important for migraine, including serotonin, norepinephrine, dopamine, and γ-aminobutyric acid *(12)*. This important relationship between estrogen and pain-modulating neurotransmitters results in increasing headache susceptibility when estrogen cycles from high to low levels (such as with menstruation), and reduced headache susceptibility when estrogen is maintained at a high level (such as with pregnancy). Variability of estrogen levels during the perimenopause period often results in migraine aggravation when women are experiencing other estrogen-related perimenopausal symptoms, such as hot flashes.

Table 5
Results of Targeted Evaluation for Patient 2:
Steven—12-Year-Old Student

Targeted assessment	Findings
History	○ Pain is across his forehead.
	○ Headaches began around age 7 without any inciting event.
	○ Pain is intermittent, with each episode lasting about 3 hours.
	○ He wants to lie down when a headache occurs, but after sleeping for 1 hour, he will awake feeling fine.
	○ No health concerns.
	○ No medications.
	○ ROS unremarkable.
Physical exam	
• Musculoskeletal	○ Normal musculoskeletal exam.
• Neurological	○ Normal neurological exam.

ROS, review of systems.

Imaging studies for headache are generally reserved for patients with traumatic or progressive headache, an abnormal neurological examination, or failure to respond to standard headache therapies. Magnetic resonance imaging scans will show small, nonspecific white matter bright spots in about 30% of migraineurs *(13)*. Interestingly, these white matter lesions have not been consistently correlated with headache duration, severity, or frequency, suggesting that they are not indicative of progressive central nervous system damage. Additionally, studies have failed to correlate these findings with neurological loss or increased risk of dementia *(13,14)*.

1.2.2. Patient 2: Steven—12-Year-Old Seventh-Grader (Table 5)

Steven reports bifrontal headaches of relatively brief duration. He endorses no associated migrainous features and has no additional neurological complaints. His examination is unremarkable. No additional testing is ordered, and he is diagnosed with migraine.

Childhood migraine is underrecognized because parents often do not realize that migraine can begin before adolescence, and headache features are often different in children compared with adults. In early childhood, about 5% of children have migraine. Peak age of migraine onset is earlier in boys than girls (age 5 versus 12 years *[15]*). In girls, migraine onset is often linked with menarche. Childhood migraine episodes are generally shorter in duration than adult migraine. In about 20% of children and adolescents, migraine attacks last less than 2 hours *(16)*. In addition, children are less likely to endorse migraine descriptors like aura, unilateral pain, throbbing, photophobia, phonophobia, and nausea on interview, although at least some of these features will be recognized in the majority of child migraineurs when diaries are reviewed *(17)*. Rather than describing sensitivities to noise and light, children may report that they "feel better" if they go to the nurse's office or lay down in bed. Asking children to draw a picture of what they feel like when they have a headache can be another effective tool for identifying migraine features *(18)*.

Migraines also tend to occur in relation to school stress, with most children experiencing headaches during the school day and being headache-free for after-school activities, weekends, and school vacations. A survey of almost 2000 adolescent migraineurs revealed that migraine most commonly occurred during school time, typically on Monday through Wednesday between 6 AM and 6 PM *(19)*. The strong influence of school stress on pediatric migraine frequently leads to the false interpretation by peers, teachers, and parents that the reports of headache are fictitious excuses to avoid schoolwork rather than a physiological reaction to school-related stressors.

As in Steven's case, neuroimaging is usually not necessary in children presenting with headaches. A meta-analysis of five studies evaluating 526 children with headaches who underwent neuroimaging identified abnormalities in 55 children, although 41 of these were incidental or nonsurgical. In the 14 children with surgical pathology (3% of the total sample), all of the children had abnormal neurological examinations *(20)*. Even in children presenting to the emergency room with headaches, imaging studies generally identify significant pathology only in children with traumatic headaches, history of a neurological disease (e.g., hydrocephalus), or an abnormal neurological examination *(21)*. As in adults, imaging studies for headaches are generally reserved for children with a traumatic or progressive headache, an abnormal neurological examination, or failure to respond to standard headache therapies.

1.2.3. Patient 3: Mr. Hillman—45-Year-Old Pianist (Table 6)

Mr. Hillman describes brief duration, excruciating, nocturnal, unilateral eye pain. During attacks, he is driven out of bed, and even engages in self-destructive behavior (hitting a book against his head). No additional testing is ordered and he is relieved to hear that he is not losing his mind, but has a typical pattern of cluster headache.

Cluster headaches are best recognized as a severe eye pain lasting less than 2 hours. Unlike patients suffering from migraine who want quiet solitude free from sensory stimuli during an attack, patients with a cluster headache are very active during their headaches, seeking lots of sensory stimuli by pacing, showering, and smoking during attacks. Cluster headaches characteristically occur about 90 minutes after sleep initiation, although daytime episodes occur in many patients suffering from cluster headaches. Attacks tend to "cluster" into nightly attacks for about 6 weeks, followed by months or years free from any headaches. These attacks characteristically occur during the spring and fall.

Table 6
Results of Targeted Evaluation for Patient 3:
Mr. Hillman—45-Year-Old Pianist

Targeted assessment	Findings
History	○ Pain is always behind his right eye.
	○ Headaches began about 10 years ago without inciting event.
	○ Pain occurs only in the spring and fall, every night for 6 weeks. Each headache attack lasts about 45 to 90 minutes.
	○ Gets up out of bed, smokes, and paces. Wife worries because he bangs books against his head during an episode.
	○ Good general health.
	○ No medications.
	○ ROS remarkable for shortness of breath related to smoking and moderate alcohol consumption.
Physical exam	
• Musculoskeletal	Normal musculoskeletal exam.
• Neurological	Normal neurological exam.

ROS, review of systems.

Medical books and diagnostic criteria often focus on associated autonomic symptoms during cluster attacks, such as lacrimation, rhinorrhea, and pupillary constriction. In the clinic, patients suffering from cluster headaches rarely endorse these features, perhaps because they are too distracted by the severity of their eye pain to worry about other bodily changes. Migraineurs, on the other hand, often do endorse tearing eyes and a runny nose. Clinicians should ask patients suffering from cluster headaches about their behavior during attacks, reassuring patients that self-inflicting pain at the location of the headache during an attack is not uncommon in patients suffering from cluster headaches, although it should be discouraged *(22)*.

Cluster headache used to be considered a "man's" headache. Although cluster headaches used to have a 6:1 male predominance in epidemiological studies in the 1960s, this dropped to about a 2:1 male predominance in the 1990s *(23)*. Researchers postulate that increased smoking and other lifestyle changes in women over the last few decades may have resulted in this change.

1.2.4. Patient 4: Ms. Inglis—35-Year-Old Homemaker (Table 7)

Ms. Inglis has a history of menstrual migraine and still gets intermittent severe headaches. She also reports daily mild headaches. Although she reports using OTC agents only 3 days a week, a review of her headache diary shows that she actually uses several doses of analgesic every day, switching among different analgesic products every 3 days. Her examinations are unremarkable and she is given two headache diagnoses: (a) intermittent migraine that results

Table 7
Results of Targeted Evaluation for Patient 4:
Ms. Inglis—35-Year-Old Homemaker

Targeted assessment	Findings
History	○ Holocranial pain
	○ Headache began in adolescence without inciting event.
	○ Initially, severe headaches occurred only with menses. For the last 3 years, she has a bothersome headache every day that lasts all day. She also gets a severe headache once or twice a week.
	○ Daily headache does not interfere with routine. Puts child down for a nap when she gets a severe headache and lies down with a washcloth over her forehead.
	○ Good general health.
	○ No prescription medications. Advil®, Excedrin®, and Tylenol®, each 3 days per week.
	○ ROS remarkable for chronic low back pain and excessive worrying.
Physical exam	
• Musculoskeletal	○ Mildly decreased cervical ROM with mild tenderness to palpation bilaterally. Normal jaw movement without tenderness.
• Neurological	○ Normal neurological exam.

ROM, range of motion; ROS, review of systems.

in once- or twice-weekly isolation in a quiet environment with a washcloth blocking out light, and (b) daily probable medication-overuse headache.

In the patient suffering from a headache, daily or near daily treatment with analgesics changes serotonin receptor activity, resulting in decreased neuronal responsiveness to analgesics and increased susceptibility to headache *(24)*. Medication overuse (previously called *rebound*) headache should be considered in all patients reporting daily or near daily headaches. Like Ms. Inglis, most patients underreport pain medication use. For this reason, the diagnosis is often missed at the first evaluation, but is identified at a later visit when a headache diary has been reviewed.

Daily analgesic use will not cause headaches to develop *de novo* in the non-headache patient; however, excessive or daily acute-care medication use will generally result in worsening of underlying headaches and the development of a chronic daily headache in patients with an underlying headache condition, especially migraine. As seen in Ms. Inglis, the usual story of medication-over-use headache is a change in headache pattern from intermittent migraine to a daily tension-type headache. Every patient reporting frequent headache should be repeatedly queried about medication overuse and required to complete a headache diary to log both headache and medication use. All acute-care medi-

Table 8
Results of Targeted Evaluation for Patient 5:
Mrs. Jeffries—75-Year-Old Hospital Volunteer

Targeted assessment	Findings
History	○ Pain is located on the right temple and forehead. ○ Migraines that put her to bed began in childhood but went away after menopause. The current headaches began about 4 months ago without inciting event. ○ Pain is beginning to affect her mood, but it does not interfere with activities. ○ Pain is constant with fluctuating severity. Pain is severe with brushing the scalp. ○ General health is fair, with treated hypertension and hypercholesterolemia. ○ ROS remarkable for low-grade fevers.
Physical exam • Musculoskeletal	○ Moderately restricted cervical ROM and diffuse muscle tenderness. Neck movements do not affect head pain.
• Neurological	○ Normal neurological exam.

ROS, review of systems; ROM, range of motion.

cations (triptans, ergotamine, analgesic or analgesic combinations, opioids, and butalbital combinations) may contribute to a medication-overuse headache. Probable medication-overuse headache should be considered in patients with benign headache taking any acute-care medication or combination of acute-care medications on a regular basis 3 or more days per week. Switching among different acute care agents on different days does not minimize the risk of medication-overuse headache. To avoid aggravation of headache by medication overuse, patients should have at least 5 days per week during which they use no acute-care medication.

1.2.5. Patient 5: Mrs. Jeffries—75-Year-Old Hospital Volunteer (Table 8)

Mrs. Jeffries reports a lifelong history of migraine, which resolved following menopause. She now describes a new-onset, unilateral pain, and low-grade fevers. She has cervical musculoskeletal dysfunction, which does not appear to aggravate her head pain, and a normal neurological examination. Because of her age and recent onset of a new type of headache, additional testing is needed. Temporal or giant-cell arteritis needs to be considered in all patients over 50 years old with a new-onset headache. The likelihood of vasculitis is high in Mrs. Jefferies owing to her age and scalp sensitivity. She was evaluated with an erythrocyte sedimentation rate (ESR) and a temporal artery biopsy. The presumptive diagnosis of temporal arteritis was confirmed by a highly elevated ESR and the subsequent biopsy.

Temporal arteritis, or giant-cell arteritis, is experienced as head pain or scalp tenderness, often associated with fatigue with chewing, visual disturbance, and low-grade fever. Temporal arteritis may also occur in patients with polymyalgia rheumatica, with head pain associated with proximal limb stiffness and weakness, fatigue, and weight loss. Temporal arteritis is a medical emergency that should be considered in the differential diagnosis of new headache in elderly patients because of the significant risk for vision loss and stroke. Visual ischemic complications occur in 26% of patients, and irreversible blindness occurs in 15% of patients with biopsy-proven temporal arteritis *(25)*. Stroke, usually in the vertebrobasilar distribution, occurs in about 3% of patients with temporal arteritis *(26)*.

Evaluation begins with a hematocrit and ESR. Patients with strong presumptive diagnoses of temporal arteritis or anterior ischemic neuropathy should be treated with steroids presumptively, immediately after blood work is obtained. A temporal artery biopsy should be performed within 2 to 3 days of initiating steroid therapy. Inflammatory changes in temporal arteritis often skip areas of the blood vessels, so a minimum of 1 cm of artery should be removed to improve diagnostic yield *(27)*.

2. TREATING HEAD PAIN

Disease-specific restorative treatments may be used to treat probable medication-overuse headache in Mrs. Inglis and temporal arteritis in Mrs. Jefferies. Treating migraine and cluster headache will necessitate long-term chronic pain management.

2.1. Migraine

Migraine treatment is determined by headache severity and frequency. Infrequent headaches (regularly occurring ≤2 days per week) may be managed by acute or flare therapy (Table 9). Analgesics (including aspirin or nonsteroidal anti-inflammatory drugs) are usually effective for milder migraines that are not disabling or associated with severe nausea. Analgesic–caffeine combination products (such as Excedrin®) provide superior relief of migraine compared with analgesics alone. In a placebo-controlled study of 72 migraineurs treating three headache episodes, adding 100 mg of caffeine to diclofenac significantly increased response rate *(28)*. One hour after treatment, headache relief was achieved by 41% with diclofenac plus caffeine, 27% with diclofenac alone, and 14% with placebo. This benefit may also be achieved by combining an analgesic with a caffeine-containing beverage (such as Motrin® plus a cup of coffee or can of cola). Severe or disabling migraines are best treated with a fast-acting triptan (sumatriptan, rizatriptan, eletriptan, zolmitriptan, or almotriptan). Most patients will respond to at least

Table 9
Targeted Treatment of Migraine

	Nonmedication	Medication
• Restorative treatment	○ None	○ None
• Preventive therapies	○ Relaxation ○ Biofeedback ○ Stress management ○ Aerobic exercise	○ Antidepressants ○ Antihypertensives ○ Anti-epileptics
• Flare techniques	○ Relaxation ○ Biofeedback ○ Stretching exercises	○ Analgesics ○ Dihydroergotamine ○ Triptans

one of three triptan trials *(29)*. Combining a triptan with an analgesic may improve both the amount and duration of headache relief *(30)*. Patients with long-lasting, severe migraine attacks may prefer DHE-45 or a long-acting triptan (naratriptan or frovatriptan). Both DHE-45 and the triptans may cause a small constriction to the coronary arteries, so they should be avoided in patients with uncontrolled hypertension, a history of heart attack or stroke, or a high risk for ischemic heart disease. Patients with frequent migraine (headaches typically occurring >3 days/week) are candidates for preventive therapies. First-line migraine preventive medications include antidepressants, antihypertensives, and anti-epileptics. Selecting preventive therapy is often based on concomitant treatment of comorbid conditions, such as depression, anxiety, or hypertension. Combining both medication and first-line nonmedication treatments (e.g., relaxation and biofeedback) maximizes headache reduction *(31)*.

Treatment of early menopausal symptoms with hormone replacement therapy may result in alterations in migraine, with an equal number of women typically reporting headache worsening or improvement *(32)*. A prospective, longitudinal study of 54 menopausal women compared headache activity before and after treatment with intermittent oral, continuous oral, or continuous transdermal estrogen replacement *(33)*. Continuous, transdermal estradiol was least likely to aggravate migraine. Exacerbation of chronic headache related to estrogen replacement may be managed by reducing estrogen dosage or elimination of an estrogen cycling product. Changing the type of estrogen may also be helpful. For example, estrone is less likely to aggravate headache than estradiol *(34)*.

Mrs. Franklin was provided with an educational flyer on migraine (Box 1). Because of the frequency of her headaches, she was initially treated with preventive therapy. She had previously been treated with an antidepressant

Box 1
Educational Flyer for Migraine

What is a migraine?

Migraine is an intermittent, disabling headache. Migraines do not cause a constant or everyday headache. A migraine is often a throbbing or pounding pain on one side of the head. The pain often affects the forehead, eye, or cheek, so many people mistake their migraines for sinus pain. Migraines usually make people less productive, and some people with migraines need to lie down. Most migraine sufferers would prefer to go to a dark, quiet room during an attack. Many people feel sick to their stomachs and some vomit with a migraine.

Migraines usually run in families. Researchers believe that migraine sufferers inherit a slight imbalance in brain pain chemicals, including serotonin, norepinephrine, and dopamine. These same chemicals are important for many other body functions, such as mood and normal blood pressure. For this reason, several medications that were designed to treat other medical conditions (such as depression and high blood pressure) also have been found to help correct the chemical imbalance of migraine.

How is migraine treated?

Migraine treatment is divided into *acute* and *preventive* therapies. Acute treatment is used to relieve a specific migraine episode, such as taking Excedrin® or Imitrex® when you have a migraine. Acute treatments work best if you take them before your migraine gets really severe. Some people get a warning before a migraine begins, such as feeling tired, getting irritable, having stomach problems, or seeing spots or zigzag lines. Using acute migraine treatments during these migraine warnings can reduce migraine pain for many people.

Acute treatments should *not* be regularly used more than 2 days per week. If you usually have headaches more than 2 days per week, your doctor will probably suggest you also use a prevention therapy. Effective prevention medications include mood elevators (such as Elavil® and Tofranil®), blood pressure pills (such as Inderal® and Blocadren®), and seizure medicines (such as Depakote® and Topamax®). Although all of these medications were originally developed for other health problems, they all correct the chemical imbalances seen in migraine sufferers and decrease the number of migraine attacks.

Nonmedication treatments are also effective migraine preventive therapies:

• Stress management
• Relaxation and biofeedback
• Lifestyle adjustments: avoid fasting, eliminate nicotine, and get regular sleep
• Regular aerobic exercise: walking, biking, swimming

Where can I learn more about migraines?

Good information about migraine and its treatment can be found at these websites:

• www.dawnmarcusmd.com
• www.achenet.org
• www.headaches.org

for migraines, which caused substantial weight gain. Owing to her continued excessive weight, she was treated with topiramate (Topamax®) to help reduce migraines and obesity. She was also advised to begin a daily walking program and scheduled to meet with a pain psychologist for training in relaxation techniques and stress management. Once the overall frequency and severity of her headaches decreased, she found that those headaches that did occur responded well to Excedrin. About once each month she would have an incapacitating migraine that responded well to rizatriptan (Maxalt®).

2.2. Migraine In Children and Adolescents

The primary goal for treating pediatric migraines is to minimize interference with development and to maximize school attendance and participation. Because of the short duration of most migraines, school absence is typically not needed. Children may need a brief visit to the nurse, particularly if they feel nauseous, but they should generally be able to return to classes within an hour after receiving treatment. School is important for social and emotional development, in addition to intellectual growth. Frequent school absence creates a sense of isolation and fear of both academic and social deficiencies, additional stressors that may further aggravate pain complaints. Family therapy will be necessary when parents are hesitant to insist on school attendance. This therapy will help parents develop strategies to ensure school participation, as well as identification of manipulative behaviors that erode parents' resolve to encourage activity normalization.

Both nonmedication and medication therapies can effectively manage chronic headaches in children and adolescents. Stress management, relaxation, and biofeedback are effective nonmedication headache therapies for pediatric patients *(35,36)*. Ibuprofen and triptans are valuable and safe acute therapies for pediatric migraine, although dose adjustments are needed *(37–40)*. Generally, triptans are administered at about half of the starting adult dose in adolescents. Nasal spray and orally disintegrating triptans may be particularly useful in children. Preventive therapy with antidepressants and antiepileptics can be helpful in children with frequent and recalcitrant migraine not responding to nonmedication therapy, although side effects must be closely monitored (especially effects on cognition, energy level, weight, and menstruation *[41–44]*).

Steven was given an educational flyer (Box 2) and attended four training sessions including biofeedback and stress management. He also began eating breakfast each morning before school and going to bed at a regular time rather than staying up to fall asleep in front of the television. His mother met with the school teacher and nurse and informed them that Steven's doctor wanted him to go to the nurse when a migraine first began for a dose of ibuprofen with a drink of cola. Steven was to return to class after 15 minutes, unless he was

Box 2
Supplemental Educational Flyer for Migraine in Kids

Do kids really get migraines?

Migraine headaches often start in childhood. About 10% of all kids get migraines. Headaches usually start in early childhood in boys and during adolescence in girls. Migraines typically run in families, so your parents, aunts, cousins, or grandparents may also remember getting headaches. You may have inherited your tendency to get migraines from them. Sometimes you are the first person in your family to get migraines.

Once you have a tendency to get migraines, many things can trigger a headache episode. Common triggers include missing meals, staying up too late, and stress. Stress comes from changes in your usual routine. Both bad changes (such as a hard math class, moving, or your parents getting divorced) and good changes (such as making a new friend, starting a new elective class, or getting a new baby brother) trigger stress changes in your body. School stress is the most common trigger for migraines in kids. Most kids find their migraines occur during school hours. This can make kids, their parents, and their teacher think the headaches may be just an excuse to get out of a tough class or homework. The good news is that many migraine treatments can block stress from triggering a migraine.

Should I stay home from school if I've got a migraine?

Your most important job is doing well in school. Just like grown-ups go to work every day, kids are also expected to do their job at school every day. You should usually be able to go to school when you have a migraine. Most migraines only last a couple of hours, so there is no need to miss a whole day of school. Have one of your parents talk to the school nurse about your migraines and give the nurse your usual treatment. Many kids will go to the nurse when they start to get a bad headache. They can take their migraine medication and practice some relaxation techniques. After 15 to 20 minutes, you should return to class.

What can I do to make my migraines better?

Your doctor can give you medications. There are also a number of things you can do to help reduce your migraines:

- Go to bed before 10 PM every night. Do not watch TV or eat snacks in bed.
- Get up at least 45 minutes before you need to leave for school and eat a good breakfast.
- Do not skip lunch at school.
- Set aside a regular time and spot to do your homework after school. Do not do homework in front of the TV.
- Get regular exercise every day. You can walk, bike, swim, or join a sports team at school.
- Spend time doing fun things with your friends. Try to minimize time alone watching TV or playing computer or video games.
- Participate in a fun after-school activity, such as a sport, the marching band, or the school newspaper.

Table 10
Targeted Treatment of Cluster Headache

	Nonmedication	Medication
• Restorative treatment	◦ None	◦ Steroids
• Preventive therapies	◦ Avoid alcohol ◦ Avoid nicotine	◦ Verapamil ◦ Anti-epileptics
• Flare techniques	◦ None	◦ Oxygen

vomiting. Steven had no more school absences and briefly saw the nurse twice during the next month for migraines. His mother helped reinforce regular sleeping and eating habits and encouraged him to become more physically active by joining the middle school track team. As is typical in many boys, Steven's migraines dissipated during his teenage years.

2.3. Cluster Headache

The intensity of each individual cluster headache attack is so severe that therapy must focus on prevention (Table 10). Most people experience mild and less frequent attacks when the cluster period first begins, with attacks becoming more severe and frequent during the middle of the cluster period. Preventive treatment is most effective when initiated at the first sign of a new cluster period. First-line preventive therapy is 240 to 480 mg of verapamil daily. Patients failing to achieve a response may alternatively try an anti-epileptic, such as valproate, gabapentin, or topiramate. In patients with infrequent cluster episodes that do not respond to preventive therapy, 10 to 60 mg of prednisone daily may be used for 1 week. One hundred percent oxygen delivered by face mask at 7 L/minute for 10 minutes may provide effective rescue therapy. Analgesics and triptans used for migraine are generally ineffective rescue therapies for cluster headache because pain relief is not expected to begin until after the usual cluster attack has already ended. Anecdotally, some recalcitrant patients with cluster headaches achieve headache prevention from a bedtime dose of a long-acting triptan, such as frovatriptan *(45)*. Successful cluster treatment typically results in reduced frequency and duration of headache episodes. The intensity of each individual headache episode, however, is typically not reduced. For this reason, reduction in headache frequency is the main target of cluster headache therapy.

Mr. Hillman was given an educational flyer about cluster headaches (Box 3) and was relieved to hear that he was not crazy and that other people get head-

---

Box 3
Educational Flyer for Cluster Headache

What is cluster headache?

A cluster headache is much less common than a migraine or a tension-type headache. Cluster headaches typically occur in groups, or *clusters*. Most people will be headache-free for months to years and then wake up one night with an excruciating pain in their eye. This pain is so severe, they usually cannot lie still, and they will pace around the room, smoke, or shower. Some people press their head against the wall or floor or even hit their head during an attack. After about 45 to 90 minutes, the pain will go away. Once a cluster has started, many people know that they will have three to four severe attacks every night for the next 6 weeks. Some people also get cluster headaches during the day.

Researchers believe that a cluster headache is caused by chemical imbalances in histamine and serotonin. Why these imbalances occur in some people and why the headaches cluster is a mystery. Curiously, most people have their clusters in the spring and fall. Unlike migraines, cluster headaches do not tend to run in families, so your family may think you are going crazy when you describe these severe attacks or they see you running around with a headache.

How is cluster treated?

When your cluster first begins, you should start taking a prevention medication. The most effective medication to prevent cluster headaches is verapamil (Calan® or Isoptin®). Your doctor will have you take this every day during your usual cluster period. If this does not work, you may need to try a different prevention medication or take steroids (prednisone) for a few days. Your doctor may also have you breathe 100% oxygen during those headaches that are not prevented. For many people, oxygen makes the individual attacks less severe. Make sure you take a small oxygen tank with you to work or while running errands if you get cluster headaches during the daytime hours.

Both nicotine and alcohol are believed to aggravate cluster headaches. Some people find their cluster attacks are less frequent when they quit smoking. During a cluster period, avoid both nicotine and alcohol.

Where can I learn more about cluster headache?

Good information about cluster and its treatment can be found at these websites:

• www.achenet.org
• www.headaches.org
• http://familydoctor.org/035.xml

---

aches just like his. He was started on verapamil (Calan®) and given an oxygen tank to keep at his bedside and take to work during his cluster period. He returned after 1 week with no improvement and was prescribed a 1-week course of prednisone, with good resolution of his headaches. He was also instructed to call the office as soon as he experienced his first attack in his next cluster so that verapamil could be started right away. Preventive therapy is generally most effective when given during the first 2 weeks of a cluster period. As in Mr. Hillman, if treatment is first initiated in the middle of a cluster period, when attacks are at their most severe, steroids are often needed.

2.4. Probable Medication-Overuse Headache

Daily or near daily acute migraine medication increases both headache frequency and severity and makes other preventive therapies ineffective. Medication-overuse headache improves only after discontinuation of the offending medication(s). Analgesics may be abruptly discontinued, whereas butalbital products and opioids should be tapered to minimize withdrawal symptoms. Regrettably, improvement typically takes about 6 to 8 weeks for most patients, with significant improvement occurring in more than 80% of patients after 4 months *(46)*. During the first month after medication discontinuation, or while tapering off of butalbital or opioids, patients may be treated with low-dose, twice daily non-ibuprofen nonsteroidal anti-inflammatory drugs or tramadol. Both of these analgesics have a low likelihood for producing medication-overuse headache. After 1 month, standard migraine preventive therapies may be initiated. Because preventive therapies will not be effective if used concomitantly with daily acute care therapies, therapies that previously failed while also overusing acute therapy may be re-tried at this time.

Headache sufferers with comorbid anxiety often overuse acute medications to help tranquilize symptoms of anxiety and to alleviate fear of severe headaches. Ms. Inglis was given an educational flyer about probable medication-overuse headache (Box 4) and encouraged to visit reputable headache websites to learn more about medication-overuse headache. She was asked to eliminate all currently used migraine remedies and was prescribed 500 mg of naproxen (Naprosyn®) twice daily, with one permitted additional dose daily for severe headache. She was advised to meet weekly with the nurse practitioner and pain psychologist to reinforce the diagnosis of medication-overuse headache, encourage avoidance of overused medications, and begin stress management and relaxation skills. Ms. Inglis was incredulous that her pain pills could possibly be worsening her headache and demanded alternative treatment. When no alternative plan was offered, she angrily challenged, "Fine. I'll try this for 1 month, but when I end up in the emergency room, it'll be your fault!" She sheepishly returned to see her primary care doctor in 4 weeks, apologizing for her earlier outburst and noting that her headaches really did not get any worse when she stopped using all of the OTC medications. "I guess you were right and they weren't really helping after all." She was also starting to notice that she no longer had headaches all the time; they now only occurred 4 days a week. She continued to work with the pain psychologist and was prescribed imipramine (Tofranil®) as a headache-preventive therapy because of her

---

Box 4
Educational Flyer for Probable Medication-Overuse Headache

What is medication-overuse headache?

If you get headaches, taking too many pain medications can actually make your headaches worse. If you get headaches most days and take a pain medication at least 3 days every week, you probably have a worsening of your headaches from the medication, or *medication-overuse headache*. These headaches used to be called *drug rebound headaches*.

Headache treatments are divided into *acute* and *preventive* therapies. Acute therapies treat the headache you have right now. When you take an acute pain or migraine pill every day or nearly every day, your brain changes its chemistry. The nerves get bored of the same pain killers and begin to ignore them. The nerves also ignore your body's naturally produced pain killers. This causes you to get more headaches. So you'll find that the more pills you take, the less they seem to help. This problem happens with all medications designed to treat a migraine episode, including prescription pain killers (Fiorinol®, Fioricet®, Stadol®, Vicodin®), triptans (Imitrex®, Maxalt®, Zomig®, Axert®, Relpax®), and over-the-counter medications (Motrin®, Excedrin®, Tylenol®). Daily or near-daily use of acute therapies also prevents headache preventive treatments from working. So sometimes the reason nothing seems to help your headaches is because excessive acute medication use is blocking the effectiveness of other therapies.

How is medication-overuse headache treated?

Everyone says, "Once my headaches are better, I'll be happy to get rid of all of these pills." Unfortunately, your headaches cannot get better until the medication has been out of your system for about 6 weeks. Your doctor will have you stop or slowly discontinue your daily medication. Over the next month, your doctor may have you take an anti-inflammatory medication (such as Aleve®) or tramadol (Ultram®) for your headaches.

Once you have been off of your overused medicine, you and your doctor will need to reassess your headache pattern. If you are still having frequent headaches, you will need to start a preventive medication. Effective headache prevention includes medications (such as Elavil®, Tofranil®, Inderal®, and Depakote®) and nonmedication techniques (such as relaxation, biofeedback, and stress management). If you now have infrequent headaches, you may be able to restart acute medications as long as you have at least 5 days each week when you do not use any acute therapy.

Where can I learn more about medication-overuse headache?

Good information about medication overuse headache and its treatment can be found at these websites:

• www.dawnmarcusmd.com
• www.achenet.org
• www.headaches.org

comorbid anxiety. Four months later, she was having two migraine episodes monthly, which were well managed with eletriptan (Relpax®) plus naproxen (Naprosyn). Imipramine was tapered off and she continued to experience infrequent, easily treated migraines.

2.5. Temporal or Giant-Cell Arteritis

Patients with temporal arteritis with visual complaints should be urgently treated with intravenous steroids (e.g., 1000 mg of methylprenisolone daily pulsed in two to four divided doses for several days). Patients without visual complaints are typically treated with 60 to 100 mg of oral prednisone daily. Headache should resolve within several days after initiating steroids. Prednisone dosage should be gradually tapered during the first month of treatment so that most patients will be taking about 40 mg daily after 4 weeks. Prednisone is maintained for about 6 to 18 months, with the dosage decreased by 10% per week, or 2.5 to 5 mg every 1 to 2 weeks to a maintenance dosage of 10 to 20 mg daily. The tapering schedule is dependent on maintenance of symptomatic control and reduction in ESR. Remember that small increases in ESR often occur during steroid tapering and should not result in increasing steroid dose if the patient remains asymptomatic. Because treatment is started before a diagnosis is complete, the treating physician must not feel obligated to maintain a full 6 to 18 months of treatment in patients for whom the diagnosis has been ruled out (e.g., negative ESR and negative biopsy). This is particularly true because of the serious adverse events associated with chronic steroid use (cataracts, glucose intolerance, osteoporosis and aseptic necrosis of the femoral head, myopathy, infection risk, etc.). Mrs. Jeffries was treated with oral prednisone with good symptomatic relief after 2 days and a successful gradual taper over 12 months.

3. SUMMARY

Headache is a common symptom associated with a wide variety of medical conditions. Most new headaches are related to infections or trauma. Chronically recurring headaches that bring patients to their primary care doctors are most commonly migraine. Distinguishing migraine from other common causes of headache requires an evaluation of pain location, duration, and associated behaviors. Daily headache diaries are helpful for identifying headache and medication use patterns. Patients must be reminded to record all headaches (not just the most severe ones) and both prescription and OTC medication use to achieve an accurate picture of their headache patterns. Most headaches can be effectively controlled using medication and nonmedication treatments.

REFERENCES

1. Tepper SJ, Dahlof CG, Dowson A, et al. Prevalence and diagnosis of migraine in patients consulting their physician with a complaint of headache: data from the Landmark Study. Headache 2004;44:856–864.
2. Schreiber CP, Hutchinson S, Webster CJ, et al. Prevalence of migraine in patients with a history of self-reported or physician-diagnosed "sinus" headache. Arch Intern Med 2004;164:1769–1772.
3. Kelman L. Migraine pain location: a tertiary care study of 1283 migraineurs. Headache 2005;45:1038–1047.
4. Marcus DA. Chronic headache: the importance of trigger identification. Headache Pain 2003;14:139–144.
5. Burton LJ, Quinn B, Pratt-Cheney JL, Pourani M. Headache etiology in a pediatric emergency department. Pediatr Emerg Care 1997;13:1–4.
6. Lewis DW, Quershi F. Acute headache in children and adolescents presenting to the emergency department. Headache 2000;40:200–203.
7. Ramirez-Lassepas M, Espinosa CE, Cicero JJ, et al. Predictors of intracranial pathological findings in patients who seek emergency care because of headache. Arch Neurol 1997;54:1506–1509.
8. Kelman L. The premonitory symptoms (prodrome): a tertiary care study of 893 migraineurs. Headache 2004;44:865–872.
9. Swidan SZ, Lake AE, Saper JR. Efficacy of intravenous diphenhydramine versus intravenous DHE-45 in the treatment of severe migraine headache. Curr Pain Headache Rep 2005;9:65–70.
9a. Marcus DA. 10 Solutions to Migraine. Oakland, CA: New Harbinger, 2006.
10. Marcus DA, Scharff L, Mercer S, Turk DC. Musculoskeletal abnormalities in chronic headache: a controlled comparison of headache diagnostic groups. Headache 1999;39:21–27.
11. Marcus DA. Migraine in women. Semin Pain Med 2004;2:115–122.
12. Marcus DA. Sex hormones and chronic headache. Expert Opin Pharmacother 2001;2:1839–1848.
13. Marcus DA. Central nervous system abnormalities in migraine. Expert Opin Pharmacother 2003;4:1709–1715.
14. O'Bryant SE, Marcus DA, Rains JC, Penzien DB. Neuropsychology of migraine: present status and future directions. Expert Rev Neurotherapeutics 2005;5:363–370.
15. Dalsgaard-Nielsen T. Some aspects of the epidemiology of migraine in Denmark. Headache 1970;10:14–23.
16. Wöber-Bingöl C, Wöber C, Karwautz A, et al. Diagnosis of headache in childhood and adolescence: a study of 437 patients. Cephalalgia 1995;15:13–21.
17. Metsähonkala L, Sillanpää M, Tuominen J. Headache diary in the diagnosis of childhood migraine. Headache 1997;37:240–244.
18. Stafstrom CE, Rostasy K, Minster A. The usefulness of children's drawings in the diagnosis of headache. Pediatrics 2002;109:460–472.
19. Winner P, Rothner AD, Putnam, DG, Asgharnejad M. Demographic and migraine characteristics of adolescents with migraine patients: Glaxo Wellcome clinical trials database. Headache 2003;43:451–457.

20. Lewis DW, Dorbad D. The utility of neuroimaging in the evaluation of children with migraine or chronic daily headache who have normal neurological examinations. Headache 2000;40:629–632.

21. Kan L, Nagelberg J, Maytal J. Headaches in a pediatric emergency department: etiology, imaging, and treatment. Headache 2000;40:25–29.

22. Blau JN. Behaviour during a cluster headache. Lancet 1993;342:723–725.

23. Manzoni GC. Gender ratio of cluster headache over the years: a possible role of changes in lifestyle. Cephalalgia 1998;18:138–142.

24. Srikiatkhachorn A, Tarasub N, Govitrapong P. Effect of chronic analgesic exposure on the central serotonin system: a possible mechanism of analgesic abuse headache. Headache 2000;40:343–350.

25. Gonzalez-Gay MA, Garcia-Porrua C, Llorca J, et al. Visual manifestations of giant cell arteritis. Trends and clinical spectrum in 161 patients. Medicine (Baltimore) 2000;79:283–292.

26. Gonzalez-Gay MA, Blanco R, Rodriguez-Valverde V, et al. Permanent visual loss and cerebrovascular accidents in giant cell arteritis. Arthritis Rheum 1998;41: 1497–1504.

27. Taylor-Gjevre R, Vo M, Shukla D, Resch L. Temporal artery biopsy for giant cell arteritis. J Rheumatol 2005;32:1279–1282.

28. Peroutka SJ, Lyon JA, Swarbrick J, et al. Efficacy of diclofenac sodium softgel 100 mg with or without caffeine 100 mg in migraine without aura: a randomized, double-blind, crossover study. Headache 2004;44:136–141.

29. Mathew NT, Kailasam J, Gentry P, Chernyshev O. Treatment of nonresponders to oral sumatriptan with zolmitriptan and rizatriptan: a comparative open trial. Headache 2000;40:464–465.

30. Krymchantowski AV, Bigal ME. Rizatriptan versus rizatriptan plus rofecoxib versus rizatriptan plus tolfenamic acid in the acute treatment of migraine. BMC Neurol 2004;4:10.

31. Holroyd KA, France JL, Cordingley GE, et al. Enhancing the effectiveness of relaxation–thermal biofeedback training with propranolol hydrochloride. J Consult Clin Psychol 1995;63:327–330.

32. MacGregor EA: "Menstrual" migraine: towards a definition. Cephalalgia 1996;16: 11–21.

33. Facchinetti F, Nappi RE, Granella F, et al.: Effects of hormone replacement treatment (HRT) in postmenopausal women with migraine. Cephalalgia 2001; 21:452.

34. Aylward M, Holly F, Parker RJ: An evaluation of clinical response to piperazine estrone sulphate ('Harmogen') in menopausal patients. Curr Med Res Opin 1974; 2:417–423.

35. Sartory G, Muller B, Metsch J, Pothmann R. A comparison of psychological and pharmacological treatment of pediatric migraine. Behav Res Ther 1998;36: 1155–1170.

36. Scharff L, Marcus D, Masek BJ. A controlled study of minimal-contact thermal biofeedback in children with migraine. J Pediatr Psychol 2002;27:109–119.

37. Lewis DW, Kellstein D, Dahl G, et al. Children's ibuprofen suspension for the acute treatment of pediatric migraine. Headache 2002;42:780–786.

38. Hershey AD, Powers SW, LeCates S, Bentti AL. Effectiveness of nasal sumatriptan in 5- to 12-year-old children. Headache 2001;41:693–697.
39. Linder SL, Dowson AJ. Zolmitriptan provides effective migraine relief in adolescents. Int J Clin Pract 2000;54:466–469.
40. Winner P, Lewis D, Visser WH, et 1al. Rizatriptan 5 mg for the acute treatment of migraine in adolescents: a randomized, double-blind, placebo-controlled study. Headache 2002;42:49–55.
41. Battistella PA, Ruffilli R, Cernetti R, et al. A placebo-controlled crossover trial using trazadone in pediatric migraine. Headache 1993;33:36–39.
42. Hershey AD, Powers SW, Bentti A, Degrauw T. Effectiveness of amitriptyline in the prophylactic management of childhood headache. Headache 2000;40:539–549.
43. Serdaroglu G, Erhan E, Tekgul H, et al. Sodium valproate prophylaxis in childhood migraine. Headache 2002;42:819–822.
44. Hershey AD, Powers SW, Vockell AB, et al. Effectiveness of topiramate in the prevention of childhood headaches. Headache 2002;42:810–818.
45. Siow HC, Pozo–Rosich P, Silberstein SD. Frovatriptan for the treatment of cluster headache. Cephalalgia 2004;24:1045–1048.
46. Rapoport AM, Weeks RE, Sheftell FD, Baskin SM, Verdi J. The "analgesic washout period": a critical variable in the evaluation of treatment efficacy. Neurology 1986;36(Suppl 1):100–101.

3

Pain in the Mouth

CHAPTER HIGHLIGHTS

• Clinical evaluation of the teeth and gums, along with X-rays, is initially used to identify dental pain.

• Conditions causing nondental mouth pain are distinguished by pain quality, constancy, and triggers.

• Symptoms and signs of temporomandibular dysfunction (such as jaw deviation and clicking) commonly occur in normal individuals.

* * *

Today, you have three new patients with a chief complaint of a pain in the mouth. Each of these patients has already seen her dentist at least once for this complaint, and dental pathology has been ruled out. Each patient was advised by her dentist to see her primary care doctor for a pain consultation. Here are the stories each patient tells your nurse:

Patient 1: Mrs. Ackerman is a 69-year-old choir director. "I saw my dentist four times in the last month for this terrible tooth pain. He found a couple small cavities and fixed those, but the pain's no better. I can't open my mouth to sing or even eat with this pain."

Patient 2: Ms. Benning is a 35-year-old receptionist. "I used to enjoy my job, but now I can't stand having to talk to people. And don't even ask about eating. The pain so unbearable and I've already lost 5 pounds. Something's got to be done!"

Patient 3: Mrs. Carter is a 40-year-old homemaker. "I know my dentist thinks I'm crazy. He keeps telling me my teeth and jaw are fine, but they're just killing me. He suggested I take a class or start some volunteer work to keep myself busy, but I know something's wrong. I've already seen four dentists and am going to keep looking until someone can fix my teeth right!"

From: *Current Clinical Practice: Headache and Chronic Pain Syndromes:*
The Case-Based Guide to Targeted Assessment and Treatment
By: D. A. Marcus © Humana Press, Totowa, NJ

Table 1
Common Causes of Mouth Pain

Disease category	Specific diseases
• Dental and structural	○ Tooth disease (e.g., caries and abscess)
	○ Gum disease (e.g., gingivitis)
	○ Sinus and bone disease (e.g., sinusitis and neoplasm)
• Musculoskeletal	○ Temporomandibular dysfunction
• Neurological	○ Neuralgia

Table 2
Differentiating Characteristics Among Common Causes of Mouth Pain

	Dental pain	TMD	Trigeminal neuralgia	Atypical odontalgia
• Pain triggers	Cold, sugar, tooth pressure	Jaw opening, chewing, yawning	Touching face, talking, chewing	Usually none
• Pain quality	Varies	Dull	Sharp, electrical	Dull, throbbing, burning
• Pain constancy	Varies	Intermittent	Intermittent	Constant

TMD, temporomandibular dysfunction.

1. EVALUATING MOUTH PAIN

Although the chief complaints and brief histories in these three patients are typical, none has provided enough information to formulate an educated diagnosis. Nondental mouth pain most commonly affects women over the age of 40. Even though each patient has the same primary complaint, differences in history and examination can provide ready clues to diagnostic possibilities (Table 1). Extracting important features to distinguish among common disorders depends on a targeted evaluation that focuses on high-yield questions and examination findings that help distinguish among the many possible causes of mouth pain (Table 2).

1.1. Developing a High-Yield Targeted Evaluation of Mouth Pain

Evaluations of patients with mouth pain should be targeted to specific likely clinical scenarios to help confirm or refute clinical diagnoses. The same evaluation principles apply to each patient regarding features in the history, physical examination findings, and the need to proceed with testing. Details of the targeted examination are outlined in Table 3. Inspect the oral cavity for obvious dental pathology and percuss the teeth. Spray the teeth and gums with cold water to identify areas of sensitivity that may represent dental disease, such as early dental caries. Patients should be asked to open their mouths wide. The

Table 3
Keys to a Targeted Evaluation of Mouth Pain

Targeted assessment	Findings
• History	○ Clarify pain location—complete pain drawing
	○ Identify pain pattern (constant versus intermittent) and triggers (e.g., jaw motion, touch, etc.)
	○ Record pain precipitants
	○ Identify additional medical conditions
	○ Obtain complete review of systems
• Physical examination	○ Evaluate teeth and gums for dental disease
	○ Musculoskeletal exam:
	▪ Evaluate the TMJ with jaw opening and palpation
	○ Neurological exam
	▪ Facial movement and sensation, plus general screen (gait and extremity strength, reflexes, and sensation)
• Testing	○ X-ray of the facial bones, sinuses, jaw, and dentition

TMJ, temporomandibular joint.

normal jaw should open wider than 40 mm (about the width of two male knuckles) with no left or right deviation. To measure jaw opening, ask the patient to open wide; the examiner should be able to insert two flexed proximal interphalangeal joints between the teeth. Patients with temporomandibular dysfunction (TMD) often have restricted opening and/or jaw deviation with opening. Jaw opening in TMD may also cause audible clicks or popping and/or complaints of discomfort.

Symptoms and signs of TMD often occur in healthy adults. For example, a large population-based clinical assessment of 4289 adults reported at least one TMD-type feature in 50% of those surveyed: joint tenderness in 5%, masticatory muscle tenderness in 12%, joint sounds in 25%, restricted jaw opening in 9%, and jaw deviation 19% *(1)*. Interestingly, pain occurred in only 3%. Therefore, an accurate diagnosis of TMD must include recognition of the full pain pattern, in addition to identifying possible joint and muscle derangements.

1.2. Applying the Targeted Exam to Each Patient

Pain drawings for each patient showed only pain in the lower face or jaw, with some unrelated chronic knee pain from osteoarthritis in Mrs. Ackerman. The results of the targeted evaluation are provided for each patient in Tables 4–6. Review each patient's findings, decide if additional testing is necessary, and formulate a likely diagnosis. Then read the following sections to compare your interpretations with the patients' diagnoses in the clinic. Note that each patient has symptoms and/or signs of TMD, including pain triggered by jaw opening or chewing, restricted jaw opening, and jaw deviation. Evaluate additional pain features to help clarify the diagnosis.

Table 4
Results of Targeted Evaluation for Patient 1:
Mrs. Ackerman—69-Year-Old Choir Director

Targeted assessment	Findings
History	○ Pain is over her right jaw.
	○ Pain is intermittent and can be triggered by touching in front of her right ear or brushing the teeth on the right side of her mouth.
	○ Pain began without trauma or other inciting event.
	○ ROS remarkable for mild hypertension.
Physical exam	
• Dental exam	○ Normal dentition and gums
• Musculoskeletal	○ Jaw opening is restricted to a few millimeters. Patient does not permit palpation of TMJ or surrounding muscles.
• Neurological	○ Patient does not cooperate with facial motion testing and refuses to allow sensory examination of the right side of the face. The general neurological screen is normal.

ROS, review of systems; TMJ, temporomandibular joint.

1.2.1. Patient 1: Mrs. Ackerman—69-Year-Old Choir Director (Table 4)

Mrs. Ackerman's evaluation shows normal dentition; however, her musculoskeletal and neurological examinations are very limited. Her refusal to permit any stimulation of the right side of her face is consistent with her complaint of facial touch triggering a severe pain. This pattern is consistent with the diagnosis of trigeminal neuralgia.

Trigeminal neuralgia is experienced as a unilateral, intermittent, electric-like jolt of pain into one or more of the divisions of the trigeminal nerve, usually over the cheek or jaw. Interestingly, pain more commonly affects the right side of the face *(2,3)*. Pain is typically triggered by activating a discrete trigger point on the face, such as with touching, shaving, talking, or chewing. Curiously, patients with trigeminal neuralgia will often sit holding the painful side of the face, possibly to prevent stimuli from activating their trigger point. Between pain episodes, some people experience a residual low level of pain over the face or jaw. Trigeminal neuralgia generally affects adults after age 40. Younger patients and patients with bilateral symptoms should be evaluated for multiple sclerosis. Although sensory loss occurs in a minority of patients with idiopathic trigeminal neuralgia, identifying sensory loss warrants evaluation with neuroimaging studies.

1.2.2. Patient 2: Ms. Benning—35-Year-Old Receptionist (Table 5)

Like Mrs. Ackerman, jaw opening is also associated with pain in Ms. Benning; however, Ms. Benning is able to permit some jaw movement and palpa-

Table 5
Results of Targeted Evaluation for Patient 2:
Ms. Benning—35-Year-Old Receptionist

Targeted assessment	Findings
History	○ Pain drawing shows pain in front of her left ear and over her left jaw.
	○ Pain is intermittent and occurs with chewing and especially yawning. Only able to comfortably eat very soft foods.
	○ Pain began without trauma or other inciting event.
	○ ROS remarkable for mild depression and difficulty initiating sleep
Physical exam	
• Dental exam	○ Normal dentition and gums
• Musculoskeletal	○ Jaw opening is slow and restricted to less than two knuckles. Jaw clicks with opening and deviates slightly to the right. Left temporomandibular joint and mandibular muscles are tender to palpation.
• Neurological	○ Symmetrical facial muscle motion and sensation. The general neurological screen is normal.

ROS, review of systems.

tion. Her normal dental and neurological examinations, along with the abnormal musculoskeletal examination, suggest TMD.

TMD pain originates from the temporomandibular joint and surrounding muscles. Pain may be experienced in the jaw, face, head, and neck. TMD pain typically improves with resting the jaw, whereas it is aggravated with jaw opening. TMD is characterized by muscle imbalance and tenderness, joint dysfunction with joint clicking, popping, or locking, and pain. Nonproblematic TMD is common, with asymptomatic dysfunction or transient pain occurring at some time in most adults. A large population-based survey identified self-reported symptoms of TMD (clicking, jaw stiffness, or pain) occurring during the preceding year in 55% of adults, with temporomandibular pain in 15% *(4)*.

1.2.3. Patient 3: Mrs. Carter—40-Year-Old Homemaker (Table 6)

Mrs. Carter's pain has persisted despite successful treatment of her abscessed tooth. Careful dental evaluation has ensured that additional dental pathology is not present. Her limited dental examination in the office confirms good dentition and gums. She experiences jaw deviation and clicking, although there are no restrictions in jaw opening or jaw pain to suggest significant TMD. Mrs. Carter is diagnosed with neuropathic oral pain or atypical odontalgia.

Neuropathic oral or orofacial pain was previously called "atypical odontalgia." This pain is generally experienced as a daily, constant throbbing or burn-

Table 6
Results of Targeted Evaluation for Patient 3:
Mrs. Carter—40-Year-Old Homemaker

Targeted assessment	Findings
History	○ Pain drawing shows pain and burning in the right lower jaw.
	○ Pain is always present and not aggravated with jaw movements or facial touch.
	○ She was treated with a root canal for an abscessed tooth 6 months ago. Follow-up visits found no active disease on dental exam or X-rays, although she continued to report pain.
	○ ROS shows increasing symptoms of anxiety and worry.
Physical exam	
• Dental exam	○ Evidence of previous dental work with no tenderness of the teeth or gums to palpation, percussion, or cold water.
• Musculoskeletal	○ Jaw deviates to left with opening, with audible click and popping sound. No reports of pain with jaw movement or tenderness to palpation.
• Neurological	○ Symmetrical facial muscle motion and sensation. The general neurological screen is normal.

ROS, review of systems.

ing pain in an area without active dental disease, and most frequently in an area of previous endodontic procedures. Two surveys of patients completing endodontic surgery identified persistent oral pain in an area with no active pathology in about 5% of patients *(5,6)*. Persistent pain was recently reported in 12% of patients after completing a successful root canal with no active disease identified on clinical or radiographic examinations *(7)*. Schnurr and Brooke reported a large series of 120 patients with atypical odontalgia *(8)*. Eighty percent of these patients were female, with a mean age of 42 years. To highlight the difficulty in receiving this diagnosis, the average time of pain prior to diagnosis in this survey was more than 3 years.

2. TREATING MOUTH PAIN

Treating trigeminal neuralgia in Mrs. Ackerman, TMD in Ms. Benning, and atypical odontalgia in Mrs. Carter will necessitate long-term chronic pain management. Disease-specific restorative treatments are also routinely used to treat trigeminal neuralgia.

2.1. Trigeminal Neuralgia

Trigeminal neuralgia is usually first treated with medication, which is initially effective for most patients (Table 7). Patients often experience pain-free periods lasting months to years, so tapering medication may be attempted after the patient has been pain-free for several months. First-line therapy is treat-

Table 7
Targeted Treatment of Trigeminal Neuralgia

	Nonmedication	Medication
• Restorative treatment	○ Rhizotomy ○ Stereotactic radiosurgery ○ Microvascular decompression	○ None
• Preventive therapies	○ None	○ Anti-epileptics ○ Antispasticity agents
• Flare techniques	○ None	○ Anti-epileptics ○ Antispasticity agents

ment with carbamazepine or phenytoin. Phenytoin is useful for patients with extremely severe pain because they can achieve an effective blood level quickly following phenytoin loading. Baclofen is also consistently effective for trigeminal neuralgia. Other antiepileptics (such as lamotrigine, valproate, oxcarbazepine, and gabapentin) may be tried in patients failing to achieve benefit or failing to tolerate carbamazepine, phenytoin, or baclofen. Over time, medication efficacy usually decreases, necessitating surgical intervention. A small, prospective study followed 15 patients who failed to respond to traditional therapy with carbamazepine, phenytoin, and baclofen *(9)*. Each patient was initially treated with the carbamazepine derivative oxcarbazepine with good early results; however, surgery was eventually required in the 12 patients who completed long-term follow-up. The mean time to pain recurrence was substantially shorter with surgery compared with medical management (28 months after surgery versus 10 months with oxcarbazepine). This study supports proceeding to surgical intervention earlier when patients fail medical therapy. Surgery is usually reserved for patients no longer responding to medications or who are intolerant to medications because pain also often recurs after initially successful surgery, and surgery is associated with a significant risk for developing facial or corneal numbness. Typical invasive procedures include rhizotomy, stereotactic radiosurgery (γ-knife), and microvascular decompression.

Percutaneous retrogasserian glycerol rhizotomy is usually initially effective, but recurrence and sensory disturbance occur frequently. A longitudinal survey of 80 patients reported recurrence in 72%, with a median pain-free interval of 32 months *(10)*. Hypesthesia occurred in 63% of patients, with painful hypesthesia in 29%. A comparable survey of 98 patients with trigeminal neuralgia undergoing glycerol rhizotomy reported no benefit in 18% of patients and pain recurrence in an additional 16% of patients *(11)*. A survey of 1600 patients undergoing radiofrequency rhizotomy likewise reported good acute relief in nearly all patients, with recurrence in 25% *(12)*.

Trigeminal neuralgia may also be treated with stereotactic radiosurgery using the γ-knife. A longitudinal study of 107 patients with trigeminal neuralgia treated with γ-knife of the trigeminal root showed initial benefit in 96%, with complete relief in 80% *(13)*. Relief occurred after an average of 3 months, with relief delayed up to 13 months in 1 patient. Pain recurred in 25% after 6 to 94 months. Repeat γ-knife surgery resulted in relief in 89% of patients, with 58% becoming pain-free. Sensory loss was high in this survey, occurring in 20% after the first procedure and 32% after the second. An analogous study compared outcomes in a sample of trigeminal neuralgia patients treated with stereotactic radiosurgery (*n* = 63) or glycerol rhizotomy (*n* = 36) *(14)*. During the study (average follow-up of about 2.5 years), pain improvement occurred for 92% with γ-knife and 86% with rhizotomy. Rhizotomy produced better immediate pain relief, although recurrence was higher for rhizotomy (45%) than stereotactic radiosurgery (36%). New facial numbness occurred in 53% after glycerol rhizotomy and 27% after γ-knife.

Retromastoid microvascular decompression cushions the trigeminal nerve by placing a pad between the trigeminal nerve near its root and nearby blood vessels. This is the preferred surgical treatment for trigeminal neuralgia owing to both good efficacy and safety *(15)*. A large study compared pain recurrence in 316 patients treated with radiofrequency rhizotomy and followed for a mean of 14 years and 378 patients treated with microvascular decompression followed for an average of 11 years *(16)*. The likelihood of recurrence 2 years after surgery was 50% after rhizotomy and 24% after microvascular decompression. Among the patients treated with microvascular decompression, 65% were still pain-free 10 years post-surgery and 63% after 20 years. Microvascular decompression is considerably more effective for patients with typical trigeminal neuralgia compared with those with trigeminal distribution pain that is not associated with clear tactile triggers or is associated with facial numbness or dysesthesia *(17)*. Decompression should, therefore, be reversed for patients with clear trigeminal neuralgia features. Microvascular decompression is also safe and effective in elderly patients *(18)*.

Outcome with different surgical procedures was directly compared in 126 patients with trigeminal neuralgia treated with either glycerol rhizotomy (*n* = 51), stereotactic radiosurgery (*n* = 69), or microvascular decompression (*n* = 33) *(19)*. Treatment assignment was based on preference of the treating clinician. Post-operatively, immediate pain relief was excellent (pain relief and no need for additional medications) for 68% of patients after glycerol rhizotomy, 65% of patients treated with stereotactic radiosurgery, and 91% of patients following microvascular decompression. An excellent outcome was achieved and maintained at 6 and 24 months, respectively, by 61 and 55% after glycerol rhizotomy, 60 and 52% after stereotactic radiosurgery, and 85 and 78% after microvascular decompression.

Box 1
Educational Flyer for Trigeminal Neuralgia

What is trigeminal neuralgia?

Neuron is the medical word for nerve. *Algo* is Greek for pain. Therefore, *neuralgia* means "nerve pain." The nerve that feels sensations from the face is the *trigeminal nerve*. There is a special type of severe nerve pain involving the trigeminal nerve, called *trigeminal neuralgia*. Trigeminal neuralgia is a pain that generally affects one side of the face around the eye, over the cheek, or into the jaw and teeth. The pain is excruciating and is triggered by touching a specific area on the face, brushing your teeth, shaving, talking, or chewing. In between pain spasms, you may have no pain or just a very mild discomfort until you touch your face, talk, or chew again. The other term for this condition is *tic doloreux*. A *tic* is a spasm. *Dolor* is the Latin word for pain. Because trigeminal neuralgia pain comes as electrical shocks, each pain spasm can be called painful tics or *tic doloreux*.

How is trigeminal neuralgia treated?

Trigeminal neuralgia is usually first treated with medications that were originally designed to treat seizures (such as Tegretol® and Dilantin®) or muscle spasms (such as Lioresal®). These medications control the pain for most people. For many people, the pain will come back months or years later. If you find that medicine is no longer controlling your pain or you cannot tolerate the side effects of the medication, there are surgeries for the trigeminal nerve that are usually helpful.

Where can I learn more about trigeminal neuralgia?

Good information about trigeminal neuralgia and its treatment can be found at these web sites:

• http://www.intelihealth.com/IH/ihtIH/WSIHW000/9339/10867.html
• http://www.achenet.org/articles/18.php
• http://www.ninds.nih.gov/disorders/trigeminal_neuralgia/trigeminal_neuralgia.htm
• http://www.tna-support.org/

Mrs. Ackerman was provided with an educational flyer about trigeminal neuralgia (Box 1) and prescribed carbamazepine (Tegretol®), which substantially reduced her pain but caused intolerable dizziness. She switched to phenytoin (Dilantin®), which was better tolerated and effectively reduced her pain episodes to infrequent. After 2 years, her facial trigger again became more sensitive and pain episodes failed to respond to increased doses of phenytoin or trials with baclofen (Lioresal®) and oxcarbazepine (Trileptal®). She was treated with microvascular decompression, with good pain relief. She continued to have her pain well controlled at follow-up 2 years later.

Table 8
Targeted Treatment of Temporomandibular Dysfunction

	Nonmedication	Medication
• Restorative treatment	○ Nighttime splint	○ None
	○ Myofascial physical therapy	
• Preventive therapies	○ Nighttime splint	○ Tricyclic antidepressants
	○ Myofascial physical therapy	○ Tizanidine
	○ Stress management	
	○ Relaxation/biofeedback	
• Flare techniques	○ Relaxation techniques	○ Analgesics
	○ Heat or ice	

2.2. Temporomandibular Dysfunction

TMD may involve both muscle and joint derangements. In most cases, symptoms improve significantly with conservative treatment and surgical intervention is not necessary. Myofascial treatments, including physical therapy and relaxation techniques, are usually beneficial (Table 8). Intraoral appliances/splints provide rapid relief, although these benefits tend to lessen over time when used as monotherapy. Combining an intraoral appliance with biofeedback and stress management provides superior long-term benefits *(20)*. Adding acupuncture or botulinum toxin injections has also demonstrated benefits in several studies *(21–23)*.

Few studies have evaluated medication efficacy in TMD. Low-dose amitriptyline (25–30 mg/day) monotherapy has been shown to effectively reduce TMD pain in small open-label and placebo-controlled studies *(24,25)*. In a long-term study, moderate-to-marked improvement was recorded for 19 of 22 patients treated with 30 mg of amitriptyline (Elavil®) at bedtime for 6 weeks *(24)*. After 1 year, however, only 10 of the 22 patients reported moderate-to-marked improvement, suggesting the need for dosage adjustment or application of additional treatment in patients requiring long-term symptom management. A single, open-label study treating patients with TMD who had myofascial pain with 4 mg of tizanidine (Zanaflex®) daily for 2 weeks also reported good short-term efficacy *(26)*.

Ms. Benning was given an educational flyer on TMD (Box 2) and prescribed a nighttime splint and a low dose of amitriptyline at bedtime to assist with pain, depression, and sleep disturbance. She returned to the clinic for relaxation, biofeedback training, and stress management skills with the pain psychologist. She discontinued chewing gum and selected softer foods that could be eaten using smaller bites. She also used a telephone headset at work rather than cradling the telephone on her left temporomandibular joint between her cheek and shoulder.

Box 2
Educational Flyer for Temporomandibular Dysfunction

What is temporomandibular dysfunction?

The *temporomandibular joints* (TMJs) are the joints in front of your ears that connect the bones on the side of the head (the *temporal bones*) to the jaw bone (the *mandible*). Movement in these joints allows your jaw to open and close. Sometimes, people have pain around this joint when the jaw moves. This pain is called *temporomandibular dysfunction* (TMD). People with TMD often notice they have limited jaw motion, their joints click and pop when they open and close their mouth, and moving the jaw is painful. Opening the mouth wide, such as when eating or yawning, may produce severe pain.

When doctors first recognized TMD problems, they mistakenly thought the problem was the joint itself. For most people with TMD, the pain is actually caused by abnormal muscle tightness and spasm in the jaw muscles that surround this joint. This type of muscle pain is called a "myofascial pain."

How is TMD treated?

TMD is usually treated like other types of muscle or myofascial pain. The jaw muscles need to be relaxed. This can be done with physical therapy and wearing nighttime jaw splints. These splints relax the muscles, stabilize the joints, and prevent tooth grinding while you sleep. Some medications, including tricyclic antidepressants (such as Elavil®) and the muscle relaxer Zanaflex® may also be helpful. Surgery is seldom needed or helpful.

Things you can do to reduce TMD pain:

- Rest the jaw. Avoid chewing gum. Avoid clenching or grinding your teeth.
- Use relaxation and stress management techniques to loosen tight jaw muscles.
- Eat small bites of soft foods. Avoid apples, bagels, thick sandwiches, tough meat, and raw carrots.
- Use a cervical pillow at night to improve sleeping posture and keep pressure off of your TMJ.

Where can I learn more about TMD?

Good information about TMD and its treatment can be found at these web sites:

- http://www.odontocat.com/angles/atmang.htm
- http://www.headaches.org/consumer/topicsheets/tmj.html
- http://www.achenet.org/articles/42.php

2.3. Atypical Odontalgia or Neuropathic Oral Pain

Patients with odontalgia need a thorough dental evaluation to ensure no ongoing dental disorder is present. Establishing the diagnosis of atypical odontalgia is essential to prevent unnecessary dental procedures and extractions. Atypical odontalgia may also be more appropriately termed "neuropathic oral pain" to signify the presumed pathology of this condition. As with other types

Table 9
Targeted Treatment of Neuropathic Oral Pain (Atypical Odontalgia)

	Nonmedication	Medication
• Restorative treatment	○ None	○ None
• Preventive therapies	○ Relaxation	○ Tricyclic antidepressants
	○ Biofeedback	○ Anti-epileptics
	○ Stress management	
• Flare techniques	○ Relaxation	○ Analgesics

of neuropathic pain, antidepressants and anti-epileptics may also reduce the discomfort of oral neuropathic pain in atypical odontalgia (Table 9). The most effective treatment is tricyclic antidepressants alone or combined with phenothiazines *(27)*. Anecdotally, anti-epileptics (such as gabapentin [Neurontin®]) may also be helpful.

Mrs. Carter was provided with an educational flyer on atypical odontalgia (Box 3) and prescribed imipramine (Tofranil®) to help both her neuropathic pain and anxiety symptoms. After several visits with the nurse practitioner, Mrs. Carter accepted her diagnosis and agreed to follow-up with her current dentist rather than continuing to seek additional dental consultations. Although initially reluctant to use imipramine stating, "I have pain. I'm not depressed!", she began imipramine and saw a marked reduction in her jaw and tooth pain after about 2 months. Six months later, she returned requesting the name of a new dentist. Her pain had returned and she was again convinced she needed more dental work. Discussion identified that she self-discontinued the imipramine after 4 months because her pain was controlled and "I didn't think or worry about it anymore." Reevaluation revealed no new problems and imipramine was reinstituted, again with good pain relief and control of anxiety. Regular follow-up visits were established to help monitor long-term treatment compliance.

3. SUMMARY

Pain in the mouth does not always originate from the dentition or temporomandibular joint. Symptoms and signs of TMD (such as jaw deviation and clicking) commonly occur in normal individuals. Indeed, each of these patients had some features consistent with TMD (restricted jaw opening, jaw deviation, or joint sounds); in only one of these patients were these features significant and related to the pain diagnosis. Careful review of pain precipitants and pain characteristics usually distinguishes among common causes of mouth pain.

Box 3
Educational Flyer for Atypical Odontalgia

What is atypical odontalgia?

Odontalgia comes from the Greek words *odont* (meaning tooth) and *algo* (meaning pain). You expect teeth to hurt when you have cavities, exposed nerves, or other damage to the teeth. This would be an expected or typical odontalgia. Tooth pain that occurs when there is no ongoing dental disease is called *atypical odontalgia*. Atypical odontalgia often occurs after dental surgery, such as a root canal or tooth extraction. Although the tooth disorder is corrected by the surgery, the surrounding nerves may become irritated and start sending pain messages. When this happens, most people mistakenly believe they still have a tooth problem.

How is atypical odontalgia treated?

First, your dentist will need to examine your teeth and probably take some X-rays to make sure you do not have tooth disease. Once you have been diagnosed with atypical odontalgia, your doctor will probably suggest that you take a daily nerve-pain-prevention medication. Several medications that were originally developed to treat depression and seizures also block pain that is caused by nerve irritation. Tricyclic antidepressants (such as Elavil®, Pamelor®, and Tofranil®) are most effective. Some people also get relief from certain anti-seizure drugs (such as Lamictal® and Neurontin®). Additional dental procedures (such as additional tooth extractions or removing dental appliances) after your dentist has found no new problems is rarely helpful.

Where can I learn more about atypical odontalgia?

Good information about atypical odontalgia and its treatment can be found at these websites:

• http://facial-neuralgia.org/conditions/ao.htm
• http://www.parkhurstexchange.com/qa/A.php?q=/qa/Neurology/2004-12-12.qa

REFERENCES

1. Gesch D, Bernhardt O, Alte D, et al. Prevalence of signs and symptoms of temporomandibular disorders in an urban and rural German population: results of a population–based Study of Health in Pomerania. Quintessence Int 2004;35:143–150.
2. Loh HS, Ling SY, Shanmuhasuntharam P, et al. Trigeminal neuralgia. A retrospective survey of a sample of patients in Singapore and Malaysia. Aust Dent J 1998;43:188–191.
3. De Simone R, Marano E, Brescia Morra V, et al. A clinical comparison of trigeminal neuralgic pain in patients with and without underlying multiple sclerosis. Neurol Sci 2005;26(Suppl 2):S150–S151.
4. Ciancaglini R, Radaelli G. The relationship between headache and symptoms of temporomandibular disorder in the general population. J Dent 2001;29:93–98.

5. Marbach JJ, Hulbrock J, Hohn C, Segal AG. Incidence of phantom tooth pain: an atypical facial neuralgia. Oral Surg Oral Med Oral Pathol 1982;53:190–193.
6. Campbell RL, Parks KW, Dodds RN. Chronic facial pain associated with endodontic therapy. Oral Surg Oral Med Oral Pathol 1990;69:287–290.
5. Polycarpou N, Ng YL, Canavan D, Moles DR, Gulabivala K. Prevalence of persistent pain after endodontic treatment and factors affecting its occurrence in cases with complete radiographic healing. Int Endod J 2005;38:169–178.
6. Schnurr RF, Brooke RI. Atypical odontalgia. Update and comment on long-term follow–up. Oral Surg Oral Med Oral Pathol 1992;73:445–448.
7. Zakrzewska JM, Patsalos PN. Long-term cohort study comparing medical (oxcarbazepine) and surgical management of intractable trigeminal neuralgia. Pain 2002;95:259–266.
8. Fujimaki T, Fukushima T, Miyazaki S. Percutaneous retrogasserian glycerol injection in the management of trigeminal neuralgia: long-term follow-up results. J Neurosurg 1990;73:212–216.
9. Pollock BE. Percutaneous retrogasserian glycerol rhizotomy for patients with idiopathic trigeminal neuralgia: a prospective analysis of factors related to pain relief. J Neurosurg 2005;102:223–228.
10. Kanpolat Y, Savas A, Bekar A, Berk C. Percutaneous controlled radiofrequency trigeminal rhizotomy for the treatment of idiopathic trigeminal neuralgia: 25-year experience with 1,600 patients. Neurosurgery 2001;48:524–532.
11. Urgosik D, Liscak R, Novotny J, Vymazal J, Vladyka V. Treatment of essential trigeminal neuralgia with gamma knife surgery. J Neurosurg 2005;102(Suppl): 29–33.
12. Henson CF, Goldman HW, Rosenwasser RH, et al. Glycerol rhizotomy versus gamma knife radiosurgery for the treatment of trigeminal neuralgia: an analysis of patients treated at one institution. Int J Radiat Oncol Biol Phys 2005;63:82–90.
13. Kalkanis SN, Eskandar EN, Carter BS, Barker FG. Microvascular decompression surgery in the United States, 1996 to 2000: mortality rates, morbidity rates, and the effects of hospital and surgeon volumes. Neurosurgery 2003;52:1251–1261.
14. Tronnier VM, Rasche D, Hamer J, Kienle AL, Kunze S. Treatment of idiopathic trigeminal neuralgia: comparison of long-term outcome after radiofrequency rhizotomy and microvascular decompression. Neurosurgery 2001;48:1261–1267.
15. Li ST, Wang X, Pan Q, et al. Studies on the operative outcomes and mechanisms of microvascular decompression in treating typical and atypical trigeminal neuralgia. Clin J Pain 2005;21:311–316.
16. Ashkan K, Marsh H. Microvascular decompression for trigeminal neuralgia in the elderly: a review of the safety and efficacy. Neurosurgery 2004;55:840–848.
17. Pollock BE, Ecker RD. A prospective cost-effectiveness study of trigeminal neuralgia surgery. Clin J Pain 2005;21:317–322.
18. Turk DC, Zaki HS, Rudy TE. Effects of intraoral appliance and biofeedback/stress management alone and in combination in treating pain and depression in patients with temporomandibular disorders. J Prosthet Dent 1993;70:158–164.
19. Rosted P. Practical recommendations for the use of acupuncture in the treatment of temporomandibular disorders based on the outcome of published controlled studies. Oral Dis 2001;7:109–115.

20. Schwartz M, Freund B. Treatment of temporomandibular disorders with botulinum toxin. Clin J Pain 2002;18(Suppl 6):S198–S203.
21. Elsharkawy TM, Ali NM. Evaluation of acupuncture and occlusal splint therapy in the treatment of temporomandibular joint disorders. Egypt Dent J 1995;41: 1227–1232.
22. Plesh O, Curtis D, Levine J, McCall WD. Amitriptyline treatment of chronic pain in patients with temporomandibular disorders. J Oral Rehabil 2000;27:834–841.
23. Rizzatti-Barbosa CM, Nogueira MT, de Andrade ED, Ambrosano GM, de Barbosa JR. Clinical evaluation of amitriptyline for the control of chronic pain caused by temporomandibular joint disorders. Cranio 2003;21:221–225.
24. Manfredini D, Romagnoli M, Cantini E, Bosco M. Efficacy of tizanidine hydrochloride in the treatment of myofascial face pain. Minerva Med 2004;95:165–171.
25. Matwychuk MJ. Diagnostic challenges of neuropathic tooth pain. J Can Dent Assoc 2004;70:542–546.

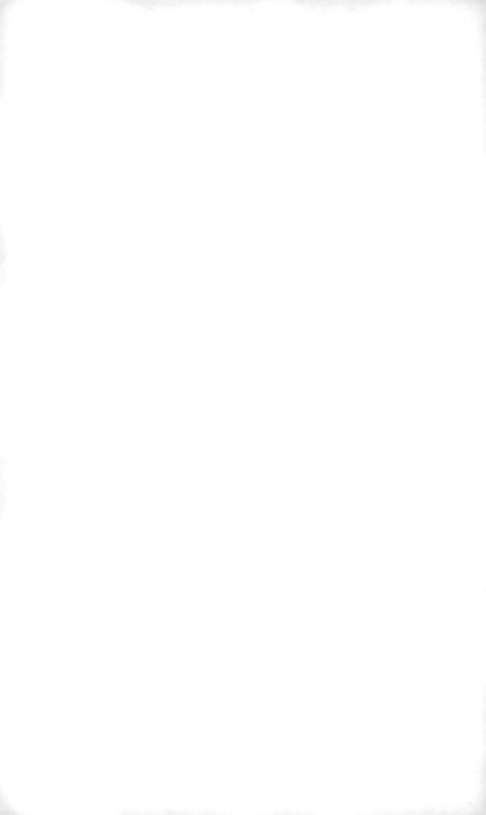

4

Pain in the Neck

CHAPTER HIGHLIGHTS

- Neck pain affects about 15% of children and adults.
- Abnormal cervical imaging studies occur in about one-third of asymptomatic young adults and the majority of asymptomatic adults 40 years of age or older.
- Risk factors for developing neck pain include stress, heavy work, prolonged neck flexion, obesity, smoking, depression, and anxiety.
- Neck pain disorders are distinguished by identifying myofascial, mechanical, and neurological abnormalities on exam.
- Musculoskeletal neck pain is effectively managed with physical therapy, acupuncture, and other pain management techniques

* * *

This afternoon, you have four new patients who range in age from 14 to 68 years old. Each patient comes to the office with a chief complaint of a *pain in the neck*. Each patient went to the emergency room over the weekend, where each was evaluated with a cervical spine imaging study. The adult patients were diagnosed with "degenerative disc disease," and the adolescent was diagnosed with "neck strain." They are all here for a follow-up appointment. Here are the stories each patient tells your nurse:

Patient 1: Mrs. Roberts is a 41-year-old obese nurse who has had pain in the back of her neck for the last 2 weeks. She attributes the neck pain to her stressful job at an understaffed nursing home. She proceeds to describe unfair treatment by an unsupportive boss and says that her husband will not help drive the kids to their numerous activities. "I keep telling my boss and husband that I need to rest. I don't know how they can expect me to get anything done with this neck pain!"

Patient 2: Miss Schmidt is an overscheduled, high-achieving 14-year-old high school student. She just returned to classes after a school break and has been under a lot of stress. After a particularly hectic day, her neck will begin to bother her. Normally, nothing keeps her from studying late at

From: *Current Clinical Practice: Headache and Chronic Pain Syndromes: The Case-Based Guide to Targeted Assessment and Treatment*
By: D. A. Marcus © Humana Press, Totowa, NJ

night, but the neck pain prevents her from bending forward to read. When she gets this pain, she just wants to go to bed. "I had this same trouble when I was in middle school. I didn't have to spend as much time studying then, so I'd just go to bed and sleep when this happened and I'd be fine the next day. Now I'm afraid I'll get behind in my advanced classes."

Patient 3: Mr. Thomas, 37 years old, has been a hard-working auto mechanic for the last 15 years. "I can't afford to miss work. I wouldn't be here, but I just can't do my job with this pain. It's so bad, I even feel unsteady when I walk in the shop. Nothing is wrong besides the neck pain. If the doctor just gives me a bunch of pain pills, I can get back to work."

Patient 4: Mrs. Underwood is a 68-year-old retired school teacher. "Since retiring, I've really slowed down. I wake up in the morning feeling like a stiff old lady. Once I get moving, I really feel more like my old self. A couple of months ago, I started painting my kitchen. Everything's fine for the first 30 minutes, but then my neck really bothers me the longer I keep painting. I should have finished painting in a couple of weeks, and now it's been a couple of months!"

1. EVALUATING NECK PAIN

Neck pain is one of the most common pain complaints heard by primary care practitioners. A survey of all patients treated in 96 general practices in the Netherlands during 12 consecutive months found an average of 33 consultations for neck symptoms per 1000 registered patients *(1)*. A Canadian survey reported an annual incidence of new neck pain in 15% of adults *(2)*. As with most types of chronic pain, neck pain is more common in women than men. A survey of three general practices in the United Kingdom identified neck pain lasting for at least 1 week in the preceding month in 16.5% of women and 10.7% of men *(3)*. In addition to gender, obesity also increased the risk for neck pain.

It is important to target specific examinations to specific clinical scenarios to help confirm or refute clinical diagnoses. Imaging studies of the spine are notorious for producing false-positive reports. Degenerative cervical disc disease—the putative diagnosis for each adult patient presented here—is commonly reported on imaging studies of the cervical spine in asymptomatic adults. Gore evaluated cervical spine X-rays in 159 asymptomatic adults (ages 20–65 years), with a follow-up X-ray after 10 years *(4)*. Although only 15% of subjects experienced neck pain during the ensuing 10 years, progressive degenerative changes were noted in 45% of subjects. After 10 years, degenerative disease was noted in the lower cervical spine in the majority of subjects (Fig. 1). When degenerative changes were noted at C5–C6, they were also typically present at C6–C7, resulting in reports of multilevel degenerative disease. Degen-

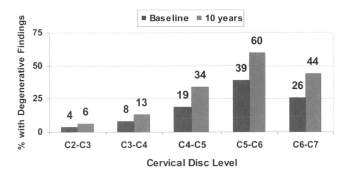

Fig. 1. Prevalence of cervical degenerative disease in asymptomatic adults at baseline and after 10 years. (Based on ref.*4*.)

Table 1
Common Causes of Neck Pain

Disease category	Specific diseases
• Musculoskeletal	○ Osteoarthritis
	○ Rheumatoid arthritis
	○ Myofascial pain
• Neurological	○ Radiculopathy
• Vascular	○ Arterial dissection
• Neoplastic	○ Focal or metastatic cancer

erative changes are most prevalent with increased age, with cervical spine X-rays abnormal in 70% of women and 95% of men between ages 60 and 65 years old *(5)*. Degenerative disc disease can be diagnosed on magnetic resonance imaging (MRI) scans in 25% of asymptomatic subjects younger than 40 years old and nearly 60% of asymptomatic subjects 40 years of age or older *(6,7)*. In an MRI study of symptom-free young adults (ages 24–26 years), MRIs identified cervical disc degeneration in 29% and disc bulges in 32% *(8)*.

Although the chief complaints and brief histories in these four patients are typical, none has provided enough information to formulate an educated diagnosis. Even though each patient has the same primary complaint, differences in history and examination can provide ready clues to diagnostic possibilities (Table 1). Extracting important features to distinguish among common disorders depends on a targeted evaluation that focuses on high-yield questions and examination findings that help distinguish among the many possible causes of neck pain. It is important to recognize that psychological distress commonly occurs in patients with neck pain. Mrs. Roberts, Miss Schmidt, and Mr. Thomas all describe high stress and worrying. Interestingly, premorbid stress,

Table 2
Keys to a Targeted Evaluation of Neck Pain

• History	○ Clarify pain location—complete pain drawing
	○ Note neck pain risk factors (stress, smoking, obesity, heavy work, prolonged neck flexion/extension)
	○ Identify additional medical conditions
	○ Record pain precipitants
	○ Obtain complete review of systems
• Physical examination	○ Musculoskeletal exam: ROM and tenderness
	○ Neurological exam: Gait and extremity strength, reflexes, and sensation
• Testing	○ X-ray of the cervical spine for mechanical signs
	○ NCS/EMG for peripheral neuropathy versus cervical radiculopathy
	○ MRI for cervical radiculopathy or myelopathy

MRI, magnetic resonance imaging; NCS/EMG, nerve conduction study/electromyography; ROM, range of motion.

depression, and anxiety all increase the risk for developing neck pain *(9)*. Although psychological symptoms serve as predictive risk factors for neck pain, this association should not suggest that the pain symptoms are emotional or fictitious.

1.1. Developing a High-Yield Targeted Evaluation of Neck Pain

Certain historical features, such as history of smoking, obesity, and work duties that require awkward postures, increase the risk for developing neck pain *(10,11)*. Interestingly, both current and past history of smoking are risk factors for musculoskeletal pain. High-risk occupations for neck pain include construction workers, nurses, and military personnel *(12)*. Occupations requiring more than 20° of neck flexion for more than two-thirds of the work day increase the risk of developing neck pain by 2.6 times *(13)*. Interestingly, frequent stress is a stronger predictor of neck pain than specific work duties. Given these data, Mrs. Roberts and Mr. Thomas can be seen as high-risk patients for neck pain owing to physically demanding work requiring awkward postures and high stress levels.

Evaluations of patients with neck pain should be targeted to specific likely clinical scenarios to help confirm or refute clinical diagnoses. The same evaluation principles apply to each patient regarding features in the history, physical examination findings, and the need to proceed with testing. Details of the targeted examination are outlined in Table 2. Neurological examinations of the upper extremities to identify motor and sensory changes suggesting cervical radiculopathy are shown in Figs. 2 and 3 and Table 3.

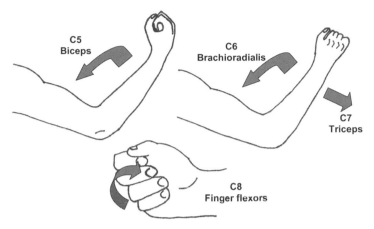

Fig. 2. Motor testing for cervical radiculopathy. Arrows denote direction of movement required to test specific muscles. Test biceps strength with palm facing up. Test brachioradialis strength with thumb pointed up. (Reprinted with permission from ref. *39*.)

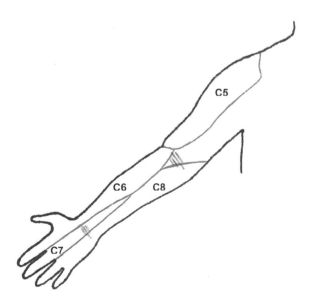

Fig. 3. Sensory distribution of cervical nerve roots. The arm is viewed from the anterior aspect, with palm facing toward the viewer. Skin areas innervated by specific cervical nerve roots are marked. (Reprinted with permission from ref. *39*.)

Table 3
Upper Extremity Evaluation for Cervical Radiculopathy

	Cervical radiculopathy			
	C5	C6	C7	C8
Motor loss	Biceps	Brachioradialis	Triceps	Finger flexors
Reflex loss	Biceps	Biceps	Triceps	None
Sensory loss	Lateral upper arm	Lateral lower arm	Middle finger	Medial lower arm
Usually affected disc space	C4–C5	C5–C6	C6–C7	C7–T1

Table 4
Results of Targeted Evaluation for Patient 1:
Mrs. Roberts—41-Year-Old Obese Nurse

Targeted assessment	Findings
History	○ Neck pain began after lifting a heavy patient ○ Pain goes into the right hand and the right middle finger tingles ○ History of a "slipped disc" in her lower back 7 years earlier
Physical exam • Musculoskeletal	○ Active ROM restricted because of pain, but she has full passive ROM when the examiner moves her relaxed neck
• Neurological	○ Right upper extremity shows reduced arm extension at the elbow, depressed triceps reflex, and numbness over the palm and middle finger. Reflexes, strength, and sensation are normal in the other extremities. Gait is normal.

ROM, range of motion.

1.2. Applying the Targeted Exam to Each Patient

Pain drawings for each patient are shown in Fig. 4. The results of the targeted evaluation are provided for each patient in Tables 4 to 7. Review the pain drawings, read each patient's findings, decide if additional testing is necessary, and formulate a likely diagnosis. Then read the following sections to compare your interpretations with the patients' diagnoses in the clinic.

1.2.1. Patient 1: Mrs. Roberts—41-Year-Old Nurse (Table 4)

Mrs. Roberts' pain began with heavy lifting as a work-related injury. Her pain drawing shows neck and right forearm pain with hand numbness. She has no mechanical neck signs, but does demonstrate neurological deficits in her right upper extremity. To help localize her neurological deficits, a nerve conduction study with electromyography (NCS/EMG) was performed.

Mrs. Roberts' NCS/EMG confirmed the clinical suspicion of a right C7 radiculopathy. A survey of patients with clinically diagnosed cervical radiculo-

A Patient 1: Mrs. Roberts – 41-year-old nurse

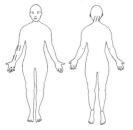

B Patient 2: Ms. Schmidt – 14-year-old student

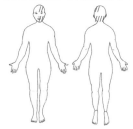

C Patient 3: Mr. Thomas – 37-year-old mechanic

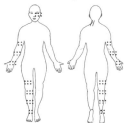

D Patient 4: Mrs. Underwood   68-year-old retired teacher

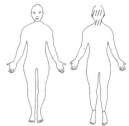

Fig. 4. Completed pain drawings for the four patients. (**A**) Patient 1: Mrs. Roberts—41-year-old nurse. (**B**) Patient 2: Miss Schmidt—14-year-old student. (**C**) Patient 3: Mr. Thomas—37-year-old mechanic. (**D**) Patient 4: Mrs. Underwood—68-year-old retired teacher.

Patients are instructed to shade all painful areas using the following key: //// = pain; :::::: = numbness; **** = burning or hypersensitivity.

Table 5
Results of Targeted Evaluation for Patient 2:
Miss Schmidt—14-Year-Old Student

Targeted assessment	Findings
History	○ Bouts of neck pain about twice a month and always with menses.
	○ When she gets neck pain and tenderness she usually tries to go to sleep. If she does, she will wake up in a couple of hours feeling fine. If cannot go to sleep, the pain will creep over her head until one side of her head is throbbing and she feels nauseated. If she cannot go right to sleep, she will usually throw up and then feel better.
	○ She rarely has bouts of neck pain during school vacations or on weekends.
Physical exam	
• Musculoskeletal	○ Full-neck ROM, with mild tenderness over trapezius muscles bilaterally
• Neurological	○ Normal screening exam

ROM, range of motion.

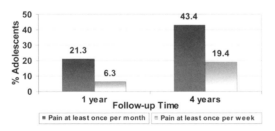

Fig. 5. Development of neck pain in adolescents who were pain-free as pre-adolescents. (Based on ref. *18*.)

pathy found EMG abnormalities in 52% and MRI abnormalities in 48% *(14)*. As expected, abnormal testing with either test was most frequent in patients with more definite clinical signs of radiculopathy, such as Mrs. Roberts. A follow-up MRI scan in Mrs. Roberts identified a right-sided herniated disc at C6–C7. Mrs. Roberts has several risk factors for radiculopathy, including obesity, heavy work duties, and a history of lumbar disc disease. A survey of 561 patients with cervical radiculopathy revealed a history of lumbar radiculopathy in 41% *(15)*. In addition, nurses comprise a high-risk group for developing neck pain. One survey of nurses identified a 12-month prevalence of neck pain of 45% *(16)*.

1.2.2. Patient 2: Miss Schmidt—14-Year-Old High School Student (Table 5)

Neck pain is fairly common in children and adolescents. A large survey of 9 to 12 year olds showed neck pain occurring at least once per week in 15% *(17)*. A total of 366 children not reporting baseline pain were followed for 4 years *(18)*. Neck pain developed in 21% after 1 year and 43% after 4 years (Fig. 5). Importantly, neck pain resolved at the 4-year assessment in 44% of children who developed neck pain at the 1-year follow-up. Painkillers were used by 28% experiencing neck pain. In addition, as in Miss Schmidt, the severity and frequency of neck pain were correlated with the occurrence and frequency of headaches.

Miss Schmidt's pain drawing shows neck and unilateral head pain. Her examination was unremarkable except for mild trapezius tenderness. Palpation of cervical and shoulder girdle muscles did not reproduce or increase pain and, therefore, did not appear to represent an important pain generator. Her pain episodes were otherwise consistent with the clinical diagnosis of migraine. Although migraine is a type of headache, it is often preceded by or associated with neck pain. Neck pain associated with migraine attacks was reported by 70% of 200 migraineurs without aura *(19)*. Physical examination may identify additional myofascial trigger points in 79% of migraineurs *(20)*. Mechanical or joint dysfunction is rarely identified in migraineurs. A survey of 13-year-old students showed increased muscle tenderness in those with migraine but not tension-type headache compared with headache-free controls *(21)*. Tenderness in the neck or shoulder was reported to occur at least occasionally in 73% of children with migraine and often in 19% with migraine compared with often in 11% of children with tension-type headache and 1% of controls.

As is common in children and adolescents, Miss Schmidt's migraines typically occur with menses and school stress. A large survey of 320 children with chronic headache showed a strong association between school and migraine *(22)*. In this study, 80% of children who had migraine without aura had significant improvement or complete relief of attacks during school breaks, such as Miss Schmidt. After-school activities were limited for only 30% of school children with migraine. Like Miss Schmidt, attacks occurred only in the late afternoon or evening in about 45% of children. Exposure to computers and sleep deficiency were also identified as significant headache triggers. Migraine attacks are typically aggravated in girls during adolescence, possibly resulting from the hormonal changes that accompany puberty, changes in sleep patterns, and increases in school stress.

Table 6
Results of Targeted Evaluation for Patient 3:
Mr. Thomas—38-Year-Old Mechanic

Targeted assessment	Findings
History	○ About 1 week after the neck pain started, Mr. Thomas noticed some tingling and numbness in his hand and dizziness.
	○ Mr. Thomas is a smoker. He is currently being treated for hypertension and hypercholesterolemia.
Physical exam	
• Musculoskeletal	○ No restrictions of active neck movement
• Neurological	○ Left eyelid is slightly drooped.
	○ Left-sided facial sensation is decreased.
	○ Pinprick is decreased in the right upper extremities.
	○ When walking, he tends to lean to the left.

1.2.3. Patient 3: Mr. Thomas—37–Year-Old Auto Mechanic (Table 6)

Mr. Thomas' pain drawing shows neck pain with numbness over his left face and right extremities. His neurological symptoms and examination localize deficits to the lateral medulla. The musculoskeletal examination is unremarkable. An MRI of the brain identified a lateral medullary infarct. In addition, a crescent-shaped high signal was noted at the left vertebral artery, consistent with a hematoma. Cerebral angiography showed narrowing of the left vertebral lumen, read as a "string sign."

Mr. Thomas' history, examination, and follow-up testing reveal a diagnosis of left vertebral artery dissection. Vertebral artery dissection may occur after neck manipulation, trauma (e.g., whiplash injury), sports or exercise, or prolonged working in cramped spaces, as in Mr. Thomas' case (23,24). In one survey of 46 patients with vertebral artery dissection, neck pain was reported by 72% of patients and headache by 50% (11). In a similar report of 26 patients with vertebral artery dissection, neck and/or head pain (predominantly occipital) were prominent features for 85% of patients and preceded the development of neurological deficits in 53% (25). Men develop vertebral artery dissection slightly more frequently than women (59% versus 41%), with a mean age at onset of 42 years (11). Hypertension, hypercholesterolemia, and smoking are all risk factors for vertebral artery dissection (11). Mr. Thomas' clinical presentation is typical for lateral medullary infarction or Wallenberg's syndrome: facial numbness, a Horner's syndrome, and ataxia on the side of the infarction, with extremity numbness to pin/temperature on the opposite side.

1.2.4. Patient 4: Mrs. Underwood—68-Year-Old Retired Teacher (Table 7)

Mrs. Underwood's pain drawing revealed neck and posterior head pain. Her history of reproduction or aggravation of pain with postural changes suggested

Table 7
Results of Targeted Evaluation for Patient 4:
Mrs. Underwood—68–Year-Old Retired Teacher

Targeted assessment	Findings
History	○ Neck pain radiates over the back and side of her head when she tilts her head in one position for a long time, such as when painting high walls or ceilings.
Physical exam • Musculoskeletal	○ Both active and passive cervical ROM are decreased. Crepitus occurs with passive ROM of relaxed neck. The paraspinal muscles are tender and palpation triggers head pain.
• Neurological	○ Normal screen

ROM, range of motion.

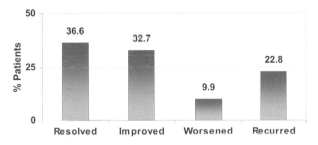

Fig. 6. Twelve-month outcome of baseline neck pain. (Based on ref. 2.)

structural pathology. Her examination showed both mechanical and myofascial abnormalities.

Review of her previously obtained neck X-ray showed several large osteophytes and disc space narrowing. She was diagnosed with osteoarthritis with cervicogenic headache. Cervicogenic headache is defined as "headache occurring with symptoms and signs of neck pain" (26). Neck pain is a prominent feature, and head pain is typically provoked by neck movements, prolonged posture, or palpation. Cervical range of motion is also typically decreased, as in Mrs. Underwood's case. Significant cervical pathology may be identified with imaging studies. Women are four times as likely as men to have cervicogenic headache, with a mean age at onset of 43 years (27).

2. Treating Neck Pain

The prognosis for neck pain is very good. Neck pain was followed for 1 year in a group of 587 adults with baseline mild neck pain (72%), high pain without disability (19%), or high pain with disability (9%) (2). Pain improved

Table 8
Treatments for Chronic Neck Pain

Effective	Ineffective
• Exercise	• Cervical traction
• Mobilization	• Soft collars
• Manipulation	
• Acupuncture (short-term only)	

Based on refs. *29–32.*

or resolved in 69% (Fig. 6). Unfortunately, pain recurred during the year after improving or resolving for 23%.

Disease-specific restorative treatments may be used to treat an acute radiculopathy and vertebral artery dissection. Mrs. Roberts was treated with conservative treatment, including physical therapy and occupational therapy, to help modify her work duties. Mr. Thomas was treated with heparin followed by warfarin. He experienced good recovery of his neurological deficits over 2 months. A prospective, multicenter study of outcome in patients with cervical arterial dissections similarly showed complete recovery of neurological deficits in 28.5% of patients, with good functional recovery in an additional 26.5% *(28)*. Treating migraine in Miss Schmidt and cervicogenic headache with osteoarthritis in Mrs. Underwood will necessitate long-term chronic pain management.

In general, physical therapy offers long-term benefits for chronic neck pain, whereas acupuncture can provide good short-term benefit (Table 8 and refs. *29–32).* Long-term outcome with physical therapy is improved by adding strength training to stretching and aerobic exercise *(33)*. In cases of myofascial neck pain, trigger point therapies, such as heat, active range-of-motion exercises, spray and stretch, transcutaneous electrical nerve stimulation, and interferential therapy, are also beneficial *(34)*. In addition, recovery from neck pain in office workers is 40% better if they are allowed to take extra breaks during their work days *(35)*.

2.1. Cervical Radiculopathy

Cervical radiculopathy is typically treated with conservative treatment if no evidence of myelopathy is present (Table 9). Surgical evaluation is indicated with an acute radiculopathy when myelopathy is present, for example, when urinary or bowel retention or lower extremity signs or symptoms are present. Surgical evaluation may also be warranted initially when motor deficits are present. A long-term outcome study for surgical treatment of patients with cervical radiculopathy showed no effect of presurgical duration of symptoms on surgical outcome until symptoms had been present for more than 48 months

Table 9
Targeted Treatment of Cervical Radiculopathy

	Nonmedication	Medication
• Restorative treatment	○ Surgical decompression if motor loss or urinary/bowel retention ○ Possibly physical therapy	○ Epidural or oral steroids
• Preventive therapies	○ Activity restrictions ○ Stretching and strengthening exercises	○ Neuropathic medications
• Flare techniques	○ Physical therapy modalities	○ NSAIDs ○ Muscle relaxants ○ Short acting opioids for severe pain unresponsive to other analgesics

NSAIDs, nonsteroidal anti-inflammatory drugs.

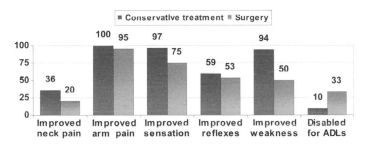

Fig. 7. Posttreatment outcome for cervical radiculopathy. Treatment was not randomly assigned, but was clinically prescribed as deemed appropriate. ADL, activities of daily living. Improved means there was complete symptom resolution or marked improvement. (Based on ref. *37.*)

(36). This study suggests that initial treatment with conservative measures in patients without myelopathy will not generally reduce the success of surgery if surgical intervention is later deemed necessary. Most symptoms aside from neck pain improve with conservative treatment in patients with cervical radiculopathy. In a survey of 119 consecutive patients with cervical radiculopathy, treatment was assigned as deemed clinically appropriate *(37).* In this sample, although arm pain and neurological symptoms improved for patients treated either conservatively or with surgery, improvement in neck pain was only modest in both groups (Fig. 7). These data support good improvement for most patients receiving conservative treatment. Improvement comparisons between

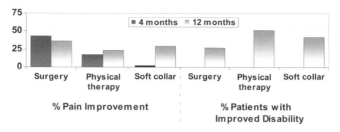

Fig. 8. Long-term outcome in patients with cervical radiculopathy randomized to surgical or conservative therapies. (Based on ref. *38.*)

conservative and surgical treatment cannot be made in this sample because patients were not randomly assigned to treatment.

A prospective, randomized study showed that surgical intervention resulted in better short-term improvement in pain than conservative treatment, although the long-term outcome was generally similar *(38).* Eighty-one patients with cervical radiculopathy without myelopathy were randomized to treatment with decompressive surgery, physical therapy (including passive modalities, traction, and stretching and strengthening exercise) for 3 months, or use of a soft cervical collar worn at least during the daytime for 3 months. Pain was assessed at baseline and 4 and 12 months after initiation of treatment. Disability was also assessed after 12 months. Although pain reduction was superior with surgery at the first posttreatment assessment, outcome was similar after 1 year (Fig. 8).

Mrs. Roberts was provided with an educational flyer (Box 1) and prescribed conservative therapy. Her exercise program progressed over 2 months from stretching exercises with passive physical therapy modalities to a home exercise program with stretches and light weights. She also worked with an occupational therapist who trained her in proper body mechanics to minimize neck and back strain while performing nursing duties.

2.2. Migraine With Neck Pain

Effective migraine prevention therapies in pediatric patients include amitriptyline, trazadone, valproate, topiramate, relaxation, and biofeedback *(39).* Effective acute-care therapies include ibuprofen and the triptans. More detailed treatment recommendations for migraine are covered in Chapter 2.

When neck pain is a significant contributor to migraine, additional therapy targeted to reducing muscle contraction may be beneficial (Table 10). For example, physical therapy including postural correction, stretching and strengthening exercises, and flare techniques is useful adjunctive therapy in migraineurs

---

Box 1
Educational Flyer for Cervical Radiculopathy

What is a ruptured disc or pinched nerve?

Nerves can be pinched when they leave the spine to go into the arm. The area where nerves are pinched is called the *root*. In Latin, *radicitus* means "by the roots." Therefore, when the root of a nerve is pinched, it is called a *radiculopathy*. When this happens, you may experience pain, numbness, and/or weakness in the arm. This is called a *cervical* (or neck) radiculopathy.

The most common causes of pinched nerves are calcium deposits from arthritis or a herniated disc. The disc is a sponge-like cushion that acts like a shock absorber between the bones in the spine. Sometimes, this sponge can shift backward or to the side, causing the nerve to be pinched. With aging, this sponge dries out and can be surrounded by calcium deposits. This causes the spaces between the bones to shrink, which is called *disc-space narrowing*. Although the smaller spaces themselves do not cause problems, this is often associated with arthritis changes that can pinch a nerve. Pinching these nerves typically results in pain in the neck and arm, along with numbness in the arm or hand. Less commonly, people develop arm or hand weakness.

How is a pinched nerve with neck pain treated?

Most cases of neck pain caused by a pinched nerve or ruptured disc improve without surgery. Standard treatments include physical therapy, muscle relaxants, pain management therapies (such as stress management, relaxation, cognitive–behavioral therapies), and pain medications. Surgery is typically used only when people have either (1) arm weakness; (2) problems with their legs, bowels, or bladder; or (3) no relief with nonsurgical treatments. Fortunately, delaying treatment for several months will not reduce the chances for surgery to be beneficial.

Where can I learn more about cervical radiculopathy?

Good information about cervical radiculopathy and its treatment can be found at these websites:

• http://www.spineuniversity.com/public/spinesub.asp?id=57
• http://patients.uptodate.com/topic.asp?file=bone_joi/8884
• http://orthoinfo.aaos.org/fact/thr_report.cfm?Thread_ID=179&topcategory=Neck
• http://orthoinfo.aaos.org/fact/thr_report.cfm?thread_id=185&topcategory=Spine

---

failing to achieve adequate headache relief from relaxation therapy *(40)*. Additional therapies that may be helpful in migraineurs with significant neck pain include the antispasmodic tizanidine *(41)*, trigger point injections *(42)*, and possibly botulinum toxin injections, although data on efficacy are mixed *(43,44)*.

Table 10
Targeted Treatment of Migraine With Neck Pain

	Nonmedication	Medication
• Restorative treatment	○ None	○ None
• Preventive therapies	○ Postural correction ○ Stretching and strengthening exercises	○ Antidepressants ○ Antihypertensives ○ Anti-epileptics ○ Tizanidine ○ Botulinum toxin A
• Flare techniques	○ Trigger-point compression ○ Local heat or ice for 15–20 minutes	○ Trigger-point injections ○ Triptans ○ Analgesics

Table 11
Targeted Treatment of Cervicogenic Headache

	Nonmedication	Medication
• Restorative treatment	○ Possibly physical therapy	○ Occipital nerve decompression
• Preventive therapies	○ Active exercise ○ Spinal manipulation and mobilization ○ TENS	○ Botulinum toxin A ○ Infliximab
• Flare techniques	○ Physical therapy modalities	○ Acetaminophen or NSAIDs ○ Occipital nerve or facet joint blocks

NSAIDs, nonsteroidal anti-inflammatory drugs; TENS, transcutaneous electrical nerve stimulation.

2.3. Osteoarthritis With Cervicogenic Headache

Cervicogenic headache is defined as "headache referred from an identified abnormality in the neck" *(45)*. Headache should be produced by neck movements or sustained neck posture. Headache may also be temporarily relieved with a diagnostic anesthetic cervical block. Cervicogenic headache is typically treated with therapeutic exercise and manual physical therapy. Most effective treatments for cervicogenic headache have only been tested in small, open-label studies (Table 11 and ref. *46*). The anti-inflammatory agent infliximab, initially infused at 3 mg/kg and repeated after 2, 6, and 14 weeks, and then every 8 weeks, provided rapid and sustained relief of cervicogenic headache in a single, open-label study *(46)*. Other headache-preventive therapies, such as antidepressants, anti-epileptics, and the antispasmodic tizanidine are also

---

Box 2
Educational Flyer for Cervicogenic Headache

What is cervicogenic headache?

Cervicogenic headache describes head pain that occurs as a result of an abnormality in the neck. The word *genesis* means "to come from," so *cervicogenic* literally means the pain comes from a problem in the neck or cervical area. Typically, cervicogenic headache is experienced as a pain in the neck that moves to the back of the head. Generally, this pain affects just one side of the head. Sometimes the pain may radiate over the side or top of the head. Cervicogenic headache episodes usually occur after moving the neck into certain positions or holding the head in one position for a long time. Often, people find that certain neck movements will also relieve the neck and head pain.

A variety of neck abnormalities may result in neck pain, with pain also in the head. These may include trauma or degenerative conditions, such as arthritis.

How is cervicogenic headache treated?

Initially, your doctor may ask you to get X rays of the neck or other imaging tests to help identify the underlying cause of your neck pain and cervicogenic headache. Ideally, the neck problem causing the head pain is treated. Often, this involves treatment of the neck muscles or joints. (For the treatment of arthritis, *see* the educational flyer in Chapter 10.) Physical therapy, including stretching exercises, trigger-point therapy, and joint mobilization are often helpful.

Where can I learn more about cervicogenic headaches?

Good information about cervicogenic headaches and their treatment can be found at these websites:

• http://www.achenet.org/articles/44.php
• http://www.achenet.org/articles/70.php
• http://www.w-h-a.org/wha2/index.asp

---

anecdotally beneficial for patients with cervicogenic headache. Surgery is reserved for recalcitrant patients with severe structural pathology.

Mrs. Underwood was given an educational flyer (Box 2) and prescribed a short course of therapeutic cervical blocks in conjunction with physical therapy manipulation and exercises. After 6 weeks, she treated her pain with a home exercise program. She also limited prolonged head tilt by purchasing a taller ladder and paint roller on a pole to reach the top of her walls. Prior to painting or working overhead, she would apply a heating pad to her neck for 20 minutes while performing neck stretching exercises. She would repeat this after activity.

3. SUMMARY

Not every pain in the neck is necessarily cervical in origin. Although each patient presented with neck pain, the cervical spine was not the origin of symptoms for every patient. A high-yield, targeted history and examination can help achieve quick and accurate diagnoses, so the next time you see a "pain in the neck" in your office, remember that neck pain may be associated with a variety of clinical diagnoses.

REFERENCES

1. Bot AM, van der Waal JM, Terwee CB, et al. Incidence and prevalence of complaints of the neck and upper extremity in general practice. Ann Rheum Dis 2005; 64:118–123.
2. Côté P, Cassidy JD, Carroll LJ, Kristman V. The annual incidence and course of neck pain in the general population: a population-based cohort study. Pain 2004; 112:267–273.
3. Webb R, Brammah T, Lunt M, et al. Prevalence and predictors of intense, chronic, and disabling neck and back pain in the UK general population. Spine 2003;28: 1195–1202.
4. Gore DR. Roentgenographic findings in the cervical spine in asymptomatic persons. A ten-year follow-up. Spine 2001;26:2463–2466.
5. Gore DR, Sepic SB, Gardner GM. Roentgenographic findings of the cervical spine in asymptomatic people. Spine 1986;11:521–524.
6. Boden SD, McCorwin PR, Davis DO, et al. Abnormal magnetic-resonance scans of the cervical spine in asymptomatic subjects. A prospective investigation. J Bone Joint Surg Am 1990;72:1178–1184.
7. Lehto IJ, Tertti MO, Komu ME, et al. Age-related MRI changes at 0.1 T in cervical discs in asymptomatic subjects. Neuroradiology 1994;36:49–53.
8. Siivola SM, Levoska S, Ilkko E, Vanharanta H, Keinänen-Kiukaanniemi S. MRI changes of cervical spine in asymptomatic and symptomatic young adults. Eur Spine J 2002;11:358–363.
9. Linton SJ. A review of psychological risk factors in back and neck pain. Spine 2000;25:1148–1156.
10. Luime JJ, Kuiper JI, Koes BW, et al. Work-related risk factors for the incidence and recurrence of shoulder and neck complaints among nursing-home and elderly-care workers. Scand J Work Environ Health 2004;30:279–286.
11. Palmer KT, Syddall H, Cooper C, Coggon D. Smoking and musculoskeletal disorders: findings from a British national survey. Ann Rheum Dis 2003;62:33–36.
12. Palmer KT, Walker–Bone K, Griffin MJ, et al. Prevalence and occupational associations of neck pain in the British population. Scand J Work Environ Health 2001;27:49–56.
13. Andersen JH, Kaergaard A, Mikkelsen S, et al. Risk factors in the onset of neck/ shoulder pain in a prospective study of workers in industrial and service companies. Occup Environ Med 2003;60:649–654.

14. Nardin RA, Patel MR, Gudas TF, Rutkove SB, Raynor EM. Electromyography and magnetic resonance imaging in the evaluation of radiculopathy. Muscle Nerve 1999;22:151–155.
15. Radhakrishnan K, Litchy WJ, O'Fallon WM, Kurland LT. Epidemiology of cervical radiculopathy. A population-based study from Rochester, Minnesota, 1976 through 1990. Brain 1994;117:325–335.
16. Smith DR, Wei N, Zhao L, Wang RS. Musculoskeletal complaints and psychosocial risk factors among Chinese hospital nurses. Occup Med (Lond) 2004;54: 579–582.
17. Mikkelsson M, Salminen J, Kautiainen H. Non-specific musculoskeletal pain in preadolescents. Prevalence and 1-year persistence. Pain 1997;73:29–35.
18. Ståhl M, Mikkelsson M, Kautiainen H, et al. Neck pain in adolescence. A 4-year follow-up of pain-free preadolescents. Pain 2004;110:427–431.
19. De Queiroz LP, Rapoport AM, Sheftell FD. Clinical characteristics of migraine without aura. Arq Neuropsiquiatr 1998;56:78–82.
20. Marcus DA, Scharff L, Mercer S, Turk DC. Musculoskeletal abnormalities in chronic headache: a controlled comparison of headache diagnostic groups. Headache 1999;39:21–27.
21. Anttila P, Metsähonkala L, Mikkelsson M, et al. Muscle tenderness in pericranial and neck–shoulder region in children with headache. A controlled study. Cephalalgia 2002;22:340–344.
22. Rossi LN, Cortinovis I, Menegazzo L, et al. Classification criteria and distinction between migraine and tension-type headache in children. Dev Med Child Neurol 2001;43:45–51.
23. Smith WS, Johnston SC, Skalabrin EJ, et al. Spinal manipulative therapy is an independent risk factor for vertebral artery dissection. Neurology 2003;60:1424–1428.
24. Dziewas R, Konrad C, Dräger B, et al. Cervical artery dissection—clinical features, risk factors, therapy and outcome in 126 patients. J Neurol 2003;250:1179–1184.
25. Bin Saeed A, Shuaib A, Al-Sulaiti G, Emery D. Vertebral artery dissection: warning symptoms, clinical features and prognosis in 26 patients. Can J Neurol Sci 2000;27:292–296.
26. Sjaastad O, Fredriksen TA, Pfaffenrath V. Cervicogenic headache: diagnostic criteria. Headache 1998;38:442–445.
27. Haldeman S, Dagenais S. Cervicogenic headaches: a critical review. Spine J 2001; 1:31–46.
28. Bassi P, Lattuada P, Gomitoni A. Cervical cerebral artery dissection: a multicenter prospective study (preliminary report). Neurol Sci 2003;24(Suppl 1):S4–S7.
29. Harris GR, Susman JL. Managing musculoskeletal complaints with rehabilitation therapy: summary of the Philadelphia Panel evidence-based clinical practice guidelines on musculoskeletal rehabilitation interventions. J Fam Pract 2002;51:1042–1046.
30. Nabeta T, Kawakita K. Relief of chronic neck and shoulder pain by manual acupuncture to tender points—a sham-controlled randomized trial. Complement Ther Med 2002;10:217–222.

72   Headache and Chronic Pain Syndromes

31. Irnich D, Behrens N, Gleditsch J, et al. Immediate effects of dry needling and acupuncture at distant points in chronic neck pain: results of a randomized, double-blind, sham-controlled crossover trial. Pain 2002;99:83–89.
32. Swenson RS. Therapeutic modalities in the management of nonspecific neck pain. Phys Med Rehabil Clin N Am 2003;14:605–627.
33. Ylinen J, Takala E, Nykänen M, et al. Active neck muscle training in the treatment of chronic neck pain in women. JAMA 2003;289:2509–2516
34. Hou C, Tsai L, Cheng K, Chung K, Hong C. Immediate effects of various physical therapeutic modalities on cervical myofascial pain and trigger-point sensitivity. Arch Phys Med Rehabil 2002;83:1406–1414.
35. van den Heuvel SG, de Looze MP, Hildebrandt VH, The KH. Effects of software programs stimulating regular breaks and exercises on work-related neck and upper-limb disorders. Scand J Work Environ Health 2003;29:106–116.
36. Kadoya S, Iizuka H, Nakamura T. Long-term outcome for surgically treated cervical spondylotic radiculopathy and myelopathy. Neurol Med Chir (Tokyo) 2003; 43:228–241.
37. Heckmann JG, Lang CJ, Zobelein I, et al. Herniated cervical intervertebral discs with radiculopathy: an outcome study of conservatively or surgically treated patients. J Spinal Disord 1999;12:396–401.
38. Persson LG, Carlsson C, Carlsson JY. Long-lasting cervical radicular pain managed with surgery, physiotherapy, or a cervical collar: a prospective, randomized study. Spine 1997;22:751–758.
39. Marcus DA. Chronic Pain: A Primary Care Guide to Practical Management. Totowa, NJ: Humana Press, 2005.
40. Marcus DA, Scharff L, Mercer S, Turk DC. Nonpharmacological treatment for migraine: incremental utility of physical therapy with relaxation and thermal biofeedback. Cephalalgia 1998;18:266–272.
41. Saper JR, Lake AE, Cantrell DT, Winner PK, White JR. Chronic daily headache prophylaxis with tizanidine: a double-blind, placebo-controlled, multicenter outcome study. Headache 2002;42:470–482.
42. Mellick GA, Mellick LB. Regional head and face pain relief following lower cervical intramuscular anesthetic injection. Headache 2003;43:1109–1111.
43. Silberstein S, Mathew N, Saper J, Jenkins S. Botulinum toxin type A as a migraine preventive treatment. Headache 2000;40:445–450.
44. Evers S, Vollmer–Haase J, Schwaag S, et al. Botulinum toxin A in the prophylactic treatment of migraine—a randomized, double-blind, placebo-controlled study. Cephalalgia 2004;24:838–843.
45. International Classification of Headache Disorders. 2nd Edition. Cephalalgia 2004; 24(Suppl 1):115–116.
46. Martelletti P, van Suijlekom H. Cervicogenic headache. Practical approaches to therapy. CNS Drugs 2004;18:793–805.

5

Pain in the Thorax

CHAPTER HIGHLIGHTS

- Screening thoracic radiographic tests frequently yields false-negative and false-positive results.
- All women 65 years of age or older and younger postmenopausal women with risk factors should be screened for osteoporosis.
- Most spinal metastases are distributed in the thoracic region.
- Antiviral and pre-emptive low-dose tricyclic antidepressant treatment of herpes zoster reduces the incidence and severity of post-herpetic neuralgia.

* * *

This afternoon, you have four new patients who are all 68-year-old postmenopausal women. Each patient comes to the office with a chief complaint of pain in the thorax that has been occurring for the last 2 to 3 weeks. They each saw a program on television talking about osteoporosis in women after menopause, and have come for a screening consultation. Here are the stories each patient tells your nurse:

Patient 1: Mrs. Thompson is a busy legal secretary who manages a large law firm. "Appearance is essential when you're the face of a busy practice. With this terrible back pain, I'm beginning to look like an old lady. I don't have time for tests and therapy. Just give me something to get rid of this pain."

Patient 2: Mrs. Underwood is a minister's wife. "This pain is really bringing me down. I can't sit still during the Sunday services anymore. Every week after services someone gives me a hug and I just want to go through the roof!"

Patient 3: Sr. Vanderhoef teaches at a Catholic college. "I feel like I'm being squeezed by a girdle. The pain was bearable until my allergies flared up. Now I'm at my limit."

Patient 4: Mrs. Wilkins is an active hiker and leader of a Girl Scout troop. "I'm just useless with this darn back pain. I've got to get this pain under control before our big camping trip next month."

From: *Current Clinical Practice: Headache and Chronic Pain Syndromes:*
The Case-Based Guide to Targeted Assessment and Treatment
By: D. A. Marcus © Humana Press, Totowa, NJ

Table 1
Common Causes of Thorax Pain

Disease category	Specific diseases
• Musculoskeletal	○ Myofascial ○ Osteoarthritis ○ Osteoporosis ○ Trauma or surgery
• Neurological	○ Neuralgias ○ Radiculopathy
• Neoplastic	○ Focal or metastatic cancer ○ Myeloma
• Infectious	○ Herpes zoster
• Endocrinological	○ Hyperparathyroidism ○ Hyperthyroidism
• Metabolic/nutritional deficiency	○ Osteomalacia

1. EVALUATING THORAX PAIN

Although the chief complaints and brief histories in these four patients are typical, none has provided enough information to formulate an educated diagnosis. Each patient has the same primary complaint; however, differences in history and examination can provide ready clues to diagnostic possibilities (Table 1). Extracting important features to distinguish among common disorders depends on a targeted evaluation that focuses on high-yield questions and examination findings to distinguish among the many possible causes of thoracic pain.

1.1. Developing a High-Yield Targeted Evaluation of Thorax Pain

Screening radiographic tests of the thoracic spine frequently yield false results. Although plain X-rays and bone scans often miss pathology, magnetic resonance imaging (MRI) regularly produces false-positive results. MRI studies performed in 90 asymptomatic adults (average age = 40 years) showed intervertebral degenerative changes and/or annular disruption in the thoracic spine in 73% *(1)*. Specific abnormalities included degenerative changes (56%), disc bulge (53%), disc herniation (37%), annular tear (58%), spinal cord deformation (29%), and Scheuermann endplate irregularities or kyphosis (38%). Interestingly, the prevalence of each of these abnormalities was similar in those adults younger and older than age 40.

Evaluations of patients with thorax pain should be targeted to specific likely clinical scenarios to help confirm or refute clinical diagnoses. The same evaluation principles apply to each patient regarding features in the history,

Table 2
Keys to a Targeted Evaluation of Thorax Pain

• History	◦ Clarify pain location—complete pain drawing
	◦ Note osteoporosis risk factors (postmenopause, low weight, inactive)
	◦ Identify additional medical conditions
	◦ Record pain precipitants
	◦ Obtain complete review of systems
• Physical examination	◦ Musculoskeletal exam:
	▪ ROM and tenderness
	◦ Neurological exam:
	▪ Gait and extremity strength, reflexes, and sensation over the thorax and extremities.
	▪ Include testing for Beevor's sign to identify lower thoracic weakness.
• Testing	◦ Blood work, as appropriate: alkaline phosphatase, phosphate, calcium
	◦ X-ray of the thoracic spine
	◦ MRI for thoracic radiculopathy or myelopathy: include saggital spine views when ruling out multiple level involvement (e.g., metastatic disease)

MRI, magnetic resonance imaging; ROM, range of motion.

physical examination findings, and the need to proceed with testing. Details of the targeted examination are outlined in Table 2. The neurological examination in patients with thoracic pain should be expanded to include sensory testing over the thorax. The dermatome for T4 circles the front of the thorax around the level of the nipples, whereas T10 covers the area around the umbilicus. Patients will also need thoracic strength testing for Beevor's sign: while lying supine, the patient is asked to raise her head, as if starting a sit-up. If there is no pathological weakness of the abdominal muscles, the umbilicus will not move. If there is weakness of the lower thoracic muscles from a spinal abnormality, the strong muscles above the umbilicus will overpower the weak muscles below, and the umbilicus will move cephalad (toward the head).

1.2. Applying the Targeted Exam to Each Patient

Pain drawings are shown for each patient in Fig. 1. The results of the targeted evaluation are provided for each patient in Tables 3–6. Review the pain drawings, read each patient's findings, decide if additional testing is necessary, and formulate a likely diagnosis. Then read the following sections to compare your interpretations with the patients' diagnoses in the clinic. Note that each patient endorses risk factors for osteoporosis in addition to age, gender, and being postmenopausal.

A   Patient 1: Mrs. Thompson – legal secretary

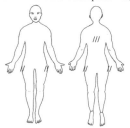

B   Patient 2: Ms. Underwood – minister's wife

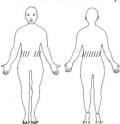

C   Patient 3. Sr. Vanderhoef – professor

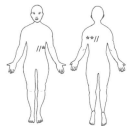

D   Patient 4. Mrs. Wilkins – Scout leader

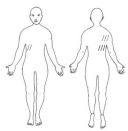

Fig. 1. Completed pain drawings for the four patients. (**A**) Patient 1: Mrs. Thompson—legal secretary. (**B**) Patient 2: Mrs. Underwood—minister's wife. (**C**) Patient 3. Sr. Vanderhoef—professor. (**D**) Patient 4. Mrs. Wilkins—scout leader. Patients were instructed to shade all painful areas, using the following key: //// = pain; :::::: = numbness; **** = burning or hypersensitivity.

Table 3
Results of Targeted Evaluation for Patient 1:
Mrs. Thompson

Targeted assessment	Findings
History	○ Risk factors for osteoporosis: began menopause at age 44, smokes 1 pack of cigarettes per day, diets aggressively to maintain slender figure, no time to exercise.
	○ Breast cancer treated 2 years ago.
	○ Pain began without trauma or other illness.
	○ ROS positive for high work stress.
Physical exam	
• Musculoskeletal	○ Restricted spine ROM. Point tenderness over her midspine.
	○ Full ROM of the hips. No tenderness to hip palpation.
• Neurological	○ Normal neurological examination, including thoracic sensation and Beevor's sign testing.

ROM, range of motion; ROS, review of systems.

1.2.1 Patient 1: Mrs. Thompson—Legal Secretary (Table 3)

Mrs. Thompson describes pain over the thoracic spine, as well as mild, bilateral hip pain with prolonged walking. Her musculoskeletal evaluation suggests mechanical spine dysfunction with no neurological compromise. An X-ray of her thoracic spine resulted in this interpretation: "Good spinal alignment. Reduction in anterior height of T7 by 30%. Remainder of thoracic spine normal."

Vertebral fractures are frequently undetected on X-rays, or the terminology used by the radiologist is not interpreted by the ordering physician as consistent with a fracture. A multinational survey assessing the diagnosis of vertebral fracture in 2451 osteoporotic, postmenopausal women compared diagnoses between local and central readers *(2)*. This study revealed a false-negative rate of 34%. In Mrs. Thompson's report, the radiologist understood that a loss of vertebral height of more than 20% is consistent with a fracture—in her case, a moderate severity fracture; however, this terminology may not be clear to clinicians reading the report. Including instructions with the X-ray prescription, such as "rule out mid-thoracic fracture," will be more likely to prompt the radiologist to render specific comments about the presence or absence of fractures than a general "screening thoracic spine" request.

Vertebral fractures may be caused by osteoporosis, osteomalacia, hyperparathyroidism, hyperthyroidism, myeloma, metastatic cancer, infection, and local trauma. Because of Mrs. Thompson's history of breast cancer, an MRI was performed as an effective tool to differentiate benign from malignant vertebral fractures. Mrs. Thompson's MRI showed normal T1-weighted signal with no gadolinium enhancement, suggesting a benign fracture *(3,4)*. Alternatively, MRIs showing involvement of multiple vertebra, gadolinium enhancement, epidural compression, or paraspinal soft-tissue masses would suggest malignant fracture *(5)*. The diagnosis of a benign fracture in Mrs. Thompson resulted in ordering bone mineral density (BMD) testing using dual-energy X-ray absorptiometry, which was consistent with osteoporosis, with a T-score less than 2.5 standard deviations below the BMD for healthy young women. The National Osteoporosis Foundation recommends obtaining BMD testing for all women 65 years of age or older and younger postmenopausal women with osteoporosis risk factors (http://www.nof.org/osteoporosis/bonemass.htm). Risk factors include older age, personal and family histories of adult fractures, thin stature, prolonged amenorrhea or early menopause, smoking, excessive alcohol consumption, low dietary calcium, minimal weight-bearing exercise, and certain medications (e.g., glucocorticoids, thyroid medications, anticonvulsants, aluminum-containing antacids, gonadotropin-releasing hormone, methotrexate, cyclosporine, heparin, and cholestyramine).

Osteoporosis affects about 6% of women between the ages of 50 and 54 years, increasing to 47% of women ages 80 to 84 years old *(6)*. Osteoporosis most commonly occurs with increased age and menopause in women; however, secondary osteoporosis may also occur with a variety of medical conditions, including endocrine, renal, gastric, and connective tissue disorders. Early life factors that predispose women to osteoporosis include prolonged amenorrhea, physical inactivity, low dietary calcium and vitamin D, smoking, and excessive alcohol use.

Vertebral fractures occur commonly in patients with osteoporosis. A longitudinal study in postmenopausal women with osteoporosis treated with calcium and vitamin D supplements demonstrated an 8% risk of first vertebral fracture within 1 year of onset of menopause, a 33% chance after 5 years, and a 55% chance after 10 years *(7)*. Most vertebral fractures are clinically silent. Hip and distal forearm fractures also occur typically with osteoporosis. Risk factors for first osteoporotic vertebral fracture in women 65 years of age or older include older age, previous nonspine fracture, low BMD, low body weight, smoking, low milk consumption with pregnancy, physical inactivity, history of falling, and regular use of aluminum-containing antacids *(8)*. Estrogen supplementation decreases fracture risk. Risk is also influenced by ethnicity. After controlling for BMD, weight, and other risk factors, a survey of nearly 200,000 American women from five ethnic groups found the highest fracture risk in Caucasian and Hispanic women, followed by Native Americans, African Americans, and Asian Americans *(9)*. Previous fractures, especially fractures associated with minimal trauma, suggest increased risk for low bone mass or osteoporosis. Failure to recognize the significance of prior fractures was highlighted in a recent survey of postmenopausal women with minimal-trauma fracture—defined as a fracture occurring while seated, recumbent

Table 4
Results of Targeted Evaluation for Patient 2:
Mrs. Underwood

Targeted assessment	Findings
History	◦ Osteoporosis risk factors: low-calcium diet, infrequent weight-bearing exercise. ◦ Good general health. ◦ One month ago, she developed a severe left-sided chest pain around her ribs and under her breast. The next day, she developed little blisters all over her left side, from between her shoulder blades around to under her breast. These crusted over in about 3 weeks, but left some scars over an area about 4 inches wide. The pain she is having now is in this same area. ◦ ROS was negative.
Physical exam • Musculoskeletal	◦ ROM testing limited secondary to pain. Patient does not permit muscle palpation.
• Neurological	◦ Gait and extremity examinations are normal. Patient does not permit sensory testing on the left thorax as a result of pain. Patient refuses to lie flat for thoracic strength testing.

ROM, range of motion; ROS, review of systems.

or standing, during normal walking, or after falling from a height of less than 4 feet *(10)*. Although half of the test subjects reported the fracture to their primary care physicians, this did not lead to counseling, BMD testing, or treatment. Another study identified a vitamin D level less than the recommended 30 ng/mL in 97% of patients hospitalized with a minimal-trauma fracture, suggesting nutritional deficiency may also play an important role in fracture risk *(11)*.

1.2.2. Patient 2: Mrs. Underwood—Minister's Wife (Table 4)

Mrs. Underwood describes, "My side feels like it's on fire. It gets worse if I go in the shower or even touch it." Her examination findings are consistent with this report. Although she markedly restricts a structured physical examination, her extreme reluctance to permit any sensory stimulation to her left thorax is consistent with a complaint of allodynia. Allodynia, a hallmark of neuropathic pain or neuralgia, is the perception of touch as pain. Touch avoidance often results in a suspicion of symptom magnification by friends, family, and health care providers, and also leads to embarrassment by the patient. Mrs. Underwood describes typical characteristics of neuralgia following an episode of herpes zoster.

Table 5
Results of Targeted Evaluation for Patient 3:
Sr. Vanderhoef

Targeted assessment	Findings
History	○ Risk factors for osteoporosis: inactivity, family history of osteoporosis with hip fracture in her mother and sister, never pregnant, daily use of aluminum-containing antacids. ○ Breast cancer treated 2 years ago. ○ Pain began without trauma or other illness, but becomes excruciating when she sneezes. ○ ROS positive for obesity and peptic ulcer disease.
Physical exam • Musculoskeletal	○ Reduced spine ROM. Mild diffuse tenderness over her thorax.
• Neurological	○ Pinprick and touch reduced below her umbilicus. Reduced vibration in both toes. Beevor's sign positive. Lower extremity testing limited owing to pain.

ROM, range of motion; ROS, review of systems.

Herpes zoster often begins with a dermatomal pain or sensory disturbance, followed within hours to days by a painful papular rash over a dermatomal distribution, which changes to vesicular and then crusted. This rash typically heals within 3 to 4 weeks. When pain persists after resolution of the rash, this is termed *post-herpetic neuralgia* (PHN). Risk factors for the development of PHN include female gender, older age, experiencing pain or sensory disturbance before the development of the rash, greater pain severity during acute herpes zoster, and larger distribution for zoster rash *(12)*. For example, 20% of patients older than 60 years of age developed PHN in a survey of patients with zoster who were treated in two clinical trials with famciclovir. This number increased to 41% when considering those patients with severe zoster pain and rash, and 47% if evaluating only female patients with severe zoster rash and pain, as well as a pre-rash pain or sensory disturbance *(12)*.

1.2.3. Patient 3: Sr. Vanderhoef—Professor (Table 5)

Sr. Vanderhoef's pain drawing shows bilateral pain, such as the "girdle" she describes in her chief complaint. Severe aggravation with sneezing explains her described link between her environmental allergies and the back pain. Sr. Vanderhoef has evidence of sensory loss and weakness below her umbilicus (around T10). She also has sensory loss in her feet, which is consistent with a peripheral neuropathy that may be related to her cancer or previous cancer therapy. Sr. Vanderhoef was also evaluated with an X-ray of the thoracic spine, which was negative. Because of her neurological deficits, an MRI scan, including a mid-saggital view, was ordered. Sr. Vanderhoef's saggital MRI scan showed two small areas of abnormal marrow signal at T6 and T9 on T1-weighted images, which enhanced with gadolinium, as well as a larger area of abnormal signal at T10. She was diagnosed with spinal metastases.

Bony metastases to the spinal column occur most frequently in patients with lung, prostate, or breast cancer. Owing to the vascular distribution around the spine, most spinal metastases occur in the thoracic region. Back pain is often the initial complaint, with later development of neurological symptoms, suggesting nerve root or spinal cord compression. A high index of suspicion is essential to prevent the development of compression of the spinal cord or cauda equina, with resultant loss of ambulatory independence. A survey of patients with malignant spinal cord compression found complaints of localized back pain and/or spinal nerve root pain in 94%, typically experienced as a band around the chest or abdomen *(13)*. Pain was generally described as severe and progressive. In 66% of patients, this pain was bilateral. As also reported by Sr. Vanderhoef, pain was precipitated in about 40% of patients by coughing, bending, and/or sneezing. One of the most significant findings from this study was the frequent and devastating delay in diagnosing malignant spinal disease in most patients. Patients typically waited about 3 weeks before reporting pain to their doctors, who typically did not diagnose their pain condition until about 3 months after symptom onset. At the time of diagnosis, only 18% of patients were still ambulating independently. Once patients lost ambulation, it was rarely regained. MRI was the most effective tool for diagnosing spinal compression. As in Sr. Vanderhoef's case, the diagnosis was often missed in plain X-rays and bone scans. In addition, plain X-rays were often ordered for the asymptomatic lumbar spine rather than the affected thoracic spine.

It is important to remember that women with breast cancer are at high risk for vertebral fracture, in addition to spinal metastases, because of changes in bone metabolism associated with cancer treatment. One study reported a 5-times-increased risk of vertebral fracture for women with breast cancer and a 20-times-increased risk in patients with breast cancer who have metastatic disease that did not involve skeletal metastases *(14)*.

1.2.4. Patient 4: Mrs. Wilkins—Scout Leader (Table 6)

Mrs. Wilkins reports pain beginning after an overuse episode. Her examination shows muscle spasm, tenderness, and trigger points that refer pain into her scapular area. There is no evidence of mechanical or neuropathic pain. Mrs. Wilkins was diagnosed with paraspinal mayofascial pain.

Myofascial pain frequently develops in thoracic muscles. Myofascial pain is characterized by tight and tender muscles with trigger points—discrete, painful muscular areas. Pressing the trigger point can result in local or radiating pain. Trigger points in the pectoral and serratus muscles often refer pain to the

Table 6
Results of Targeted Evaluation for Patient 4:
Mrs. Wilkins

Targeted assessment	Findings
History	○ Risk factors for osteoporosis: slender build, hates milk products, but drinks one glass of calcium-fortified juice each morning.
	○ Mild hypertension and hypercholesterolemia controlled with medications and diet.
	○ In preparation for summer camp, Mrs. Wilkins lifted several canoes from the ground to overhead racks, which required side bends and twisting of the back.
	○ ROS was negative.
Physical exam	
• Musculoskeletal	○ Mildly decreased ROM. Increased muscle bulk noticed on right side of spine. Enlarged muscle is tight and tender. Pressing a discrete spot on the muscle near the spine by the lower margin of the ribs causes a pain to shoot up the back and into the right shoulder blade.
• Neurological	○ Normal neurological examination, including thoracic sensation and Beevor's sign testing.

ROM, range of motion; ROS, review of systems.

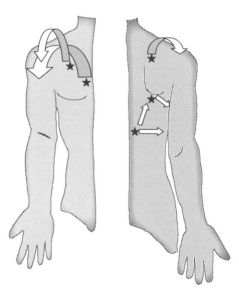

Fig. 2. Common thoracic myofascial trigger points and referral patterns. Trigger-point areas are noted with stars. Typical referral from each trigger point is shown with arrows.

arm (Fig. 2). As seen in Mrs. Wilkins, paraspinal trigger points (such as trigger points in the iliocostalis thoracis) often refer pain up the back and to the front of the thorax in a nondermatomal pattern.

2. TREATING THORACIC PAIN

Disease-specific restorative treatments may be used to treat spinal metastases for Sr. Vanderhoef. Spinal metastases from either breast or prostate cancer are treated with radiation, hormone therapy, chemotherapy, and bisphosphonates to inhibit osteolytic activity of bony metastases *(15,16)*. Sr. Vanderhoef was treated with zoledronate (Zometa®) infusion, the most effective infused bisphosphonate for women with advanced breast cancer, in addition to her other oncology therapy *(17)*. Biphosphonates are also recommended for the prevention and treatment of bone loss in patients with breast cancer who are at high risk for osteoporosis owing to hormonal therapy, chemotherapy, and treatment-induced premature ovarian failure *(18)*. Treating osteoporosis in Mrs. Thompson, PHN in Mrs. Underwood, and myofascial pain in Mrs. Wilkins will necessitate long-term chronic pain management.

2.1. Osteoporosis

Women infrequently consume adequate calcium and vitamin D, even when using supplements. A recent survey of more than 1500 women receiving screening mammograms found that adequate calcium and vitamin D intake was achieved by only 30% of pre-menopausal and 25% of postmenopausal women *(19)*. Individuals at risk for osteoporosis should be supplemented with 700 to 800 mg of calcium plus 400 to 800 IU of vitamin D *(20)*. Calcium citrate is better absorbed than calcium carbonate. Nasal calcitonin also helps increase BMD, decrease vertebral fracture risk, and decrease vertebral fracture pain. Tai Chi and weight-bearing exercise using weighted vests also improve BMD *(21,22)*.

Vertebral fractures can be effectively prevented and/or treated with a variety of medications, including oral bisphosphonates (alendronate, risedronate, ibandronate), oral selective estrogen receptor modulators (raloxifene), and subcutaneous recombinant parathyroid hormone (teriparatide) *(see* Table 7 and ref. *23)*. Clinical trials demonstrating efficacy with each of these therapies additionally treated patients with calcium and/or vitamin D supplementation. Among these treatments, bisphosphonates also significantly reduce the risk for nonvertebral fractures. Teriparatide is typically reserved for patients with severe osteoporosis and fracture risk or patients with glucocorticoid-induced osteoporosis requiring long-term steroid treatment *(24)*. Teriparatide is not recommended for use for more than 2 years, when therapy is often switched to a bisphosphonate. Teriparatide is not used concomitantly with bisphosphonates. A 3-year study evaluated the occurrence of new vertebral fractures in 1802 ambulatory, postmenopausal women with a prior fracture who were supple-

Table 7
Targeted Treatment of Osteoporosis

	Nonmedication	Medication
• Restorative treatment	○ Weight-bearing exercise ○ Muscle strengthening exercise	○ Alendronate ○ Risedronate ○ Ibandronate ○ Raloxifen ○ Calcitonin
• Preventive therapies	○ Diet with 1200 mg or more calcium/day ○ Avoidance of cigarettes and excessive caffeine ○ Limit alcoholic drinks to 1 or less/day for women and 2 or less/day for men ○ Weight-bearing exercise ○ Muscle strengthening exercise	○ Calcium ○ Vitamin D ○ Alendronate ○ Risedronate ○ Ibandronate ○ Raloxifen
• Flare techniques	○ Physical therapy modalities ○ Relaxation techniques	○ Analgesics

mented with calcium and treated with 5 mg of risedronate or placebo daily *(25)*. Women treated with risedronate experienced a 44% reduction in the risk for new fractures compared with those treated with placebo. A comparative study evaluating efficacy and cost of osteoporosis treatment in high-risk patients with low BMD and a prior history of vertebral fracture showed risedronate to be more effective and less expensive than alendronate and raloxifene *(26)*.

Mrs. Underwood was diagnosed with an osteoporotic vertebral fracture. She was prescribed 35 mg of risedronate (Actonel®) weekly, in addition to calcium and vitamin D supplements. She was also advised to begin a daily walking program. Mrs. Underwood returned to the clinic in 3 weeks, reporting that she was thinking about beginning her exercise program in a few weeks, when her work schedule might lighten up a bit. She could never seem to remember to take her risedronate until after she had already eaten breakfast, so she had not actually started it yet. She also had not taken any calcium and vitamin D ("I really hate taking pills."). At this point, Mrs. Underwood was provided with an educational flyer about osteoporosis (Box 1) and scheduled for a consultation with the nurse practitioner to review the importance of treatment compliance. At the consultation visit, Mrs. Underwood noted that she religiously followed her work schedule, but tended not to make time for herself outside of work. The nurse practitioner prescribed 150 mg of ibandronate (Boniva®) once a month to minimize noncompliance, and also recommended chocolate calcium and vitamin D chews (Viactiv®) to keep on her desk and include with scheduled healthy snacks twice daily. Finally, she was advised to arrive at the office 30 minutes early each morning and take a walk on the trails in the neighboring park before starting her work day. A co-worker joined Mrs. Underwood, which improved compliance with her walking program. Three weeks after staring this walking program, she

---

Box 1
Educational Flyer for Osteoporosis

What is osteoporosis?

Bones grow and thicken as we age and exercise them, just like our muscles. Adults usually achieve their peak bone thickness around ages 20 to 30 years. After middle age, the bones can become thinner and more brittle. Mild bone thinning is called *osteopenia*, whereas more severe bone thinning is called *osteoporosis*. (These terms come from Latin words *os*, meaning "bone"; *penuria*, meaning "lack or want"; and *porus*, meaning "hole".) Bone thinning occurs with aging, inactivity, menopause, and several medical conditions. Women with low estrogen are also at risk for osteoporosis, and menopause is a well-known risk factor. Fat cells also increase your estrogen stores, so being very thin is another osteoporosis risk factor. Osteoporosis can also occur in men. Osteoporosis is important because bones become brittle and more prone to injury when they are thin. This can cause bone fractures, even after very mild or no trauma.

Bone thickness is usually measured with a bone density scan. The dual energy X-ray absorptiometry is a common test for measuring bone thickness in the spine, hips, and wrist. This test gives you two scores: a T-score and a Z-score. The T-score compares your bone thickness to the thickness of a healthy 30-year-old. The T-score shows how much bone mass you have lost since age 30. The Z-score compares your bone thickness to the bone thickness of other people your same age. Doctors use the T-score to decide if you have osteoporosis. A negative number means you have lost bone. A T-score that is a positive number to -1 is considered normal. A T-score between -1 and -2.5 shows osteopenia. A T-score lower than -2.5 means you have osteoporosis.

How is osteoporosis treated?

The best way to manage osteoporosis is to prevent it. Everyone should eat a diet rich in vitamins and minerals to make bones strong. This should include calcium, magnesium, and vitamin D. Exercise is also important to maintain strong bones. Walking and exercises using light weights are good for bone health.

People with osteoporosis are typically treated with 700 to 800 mg of calcium and 400 to 800 IU of vitamin D daily. Additional medications that help improve bone strength are: Actonel®, Boniva®, Calcimar®, Evista®, Forteo®, Fosamax®, and Miacalcin®. These medications work to help strengthen bones and reduce the risk for fractures.

Where can I learn more about osteoporosis?

Good information about osteoporosis and its treatment can be found at these websites:

• http://familydoctor.org/136.xml
• http://www.nof.org/
• http://www.cdc.gov/nccdphp/dnpa/bonehealth/

---

began carrying 1-pound weights in her hands during her walks. In addition to improvement in her back pain, she also reported resolution of the hip pain, which was likely caused by muscular and joint deconditioning. Maintenance of benefits

Table 8
Targeted Treatment of Post-Herpetic Neuralgia

	Nonmedication	Medication
• Restorative treatment	∘ None	∘ Tricyclic antidepressants ∘ Gabapentin, pregabalin ∘ 5% Lidocaine patch
• Preventive therapies	∘ None	∘ Antiviral during zoster ∘ Pre-emptive tricyclic antidepressant during zoster
• Flare techniques	∘ Relaxation techniques	∘ Analgesics, including opioids

from a single dose of intravenous zoledronate for more than 1 year in a phase II clinical study led to phase III trials currently underway, which may result in a once-yearly bisphosphonate infusion as an osteoporosis-preventive therapy option in some patients to maximize compliance *(27)*.

2.2. Post-Herpetic Neuralgia

The incidence and severity of PHN may be reduced in patients treated with antiviral therapies during the acute herpes zoster episode, with the best reduction found with famciclovir and valacyclovir use, and slightly less of a reduction found with acyclovir use *(28,29)*. Despite adequate antiviral treatment during the first 72 hours of onset of herpes zoster, however, about 20% of adults over 50 years old will develop PHN that persists for at least 6 months. Anecdotally, the addition of pre-emptive tricyclic antidepressants, gabapentin, or opioid analgesics during the acute treatment of herpes zoster may also reduce the risk and severity of PHN. A controlled study randomized 72 patients with herpes zoster diagnosed within 48 hours of rash onset to either 25 mg of amitriptyline or placebo daily for 3 months. After 6 months, 84% treated with amitriptyline were pain-free compared with 65% treated with placebo *(30)*. In a recent rodent study, PHN was suppressed following administration of gabapentin after inoculation with herpes virus resulted in zoster lesions *(31)*. Local or topical lidocaine does not prevent PHN *(32)*. Although corticosteroids may reduce the severity and duration of zoster, they do not reduce PHN. The American Academy of Neurology recommends tricyclic antidepressants (amitriptyline, nortriptyline, maproltiline, and despiramine), anti-epileptics (gabapentin and pregabalin), lidocaine patches, and opioids (controlled-release oxycodone or morphine) as first-line therapies for PHN (*see* Table 8 and ref. *33*). Nortriptyline and despiramine are preferred because of superior tolerability. Second-line treatments include capcaisin cream, aspirin cream, and tramadol.

Box 2
Educational Flyer for Post-Herpetic Neuralgia

What is post-herpetic neuralgia?

Herpes viruses cause rashes with little vesicles or blisters, including chickenpox. After someone has chickenpox, the virus stays inactive in the nervous system. After age 50, the virus may become active again, causing another very painful rash that usually forms a band. This new rash is called *herpes zoster*. (*Zoster* is the Greek word for girdle or belt because this rash often goes around one side of the trunk or back.) In most people, the pain goes away as the rash crusts over and resolves, usually in about 3 weeks. In about 20% of people, pain may persist for weeks, months, or years after the rash has gone. This persistent pain over the area where you had the zoster rash is called *post-herpetic neuralgia* (which means you have nerve pain after the herpes infection). You are more likely to get post-herpetic neuralgia if you are older. For example, after age 70, almost 75% of people with zoster rashes will develop post-herpetic neuralgia.

How is post-herpetic neuralgia treated?

As soon as you develop a zoster rash, see your doctor to start anti-viral medications. Tricyclic antidepressant medications are very effective for neuralgia pain, and can help reduce your risk of developing post-herpetic neuralgia if you take them once the rash begins.

If you still have pain once the zoster rash is gone, your doctor may treat you with medications for nerve pain. Nerve pain medications include tricyclic antidepressants (such as Elavil®, Pamelor®, and Norpramin®) and some medications that also treat seizures or epilepsy (including Neurontin® and Lyrica®). Your doctor may also ask you to wear a patch that contains a numbing medicine lidocaine (Lidoderm® patch). Sometimes, capcaisin (Zostrix®), the ingredient in hot peppers that makes them burn, is rubbed several times daily over the painful area. Pain killers may also be needed.

Where can I learn more about post-herpetic neuralgia?

Good information about post-herpetic neuralgia and its treatment can be found at these websites:

• http://familydoctor.org/574.xml
• http://www.vzvfoundation.org/
• http://www.aftershingles.com/phn.html
• http://www.mayoclinic.com/invoke.cfm?id=DS00277

Mrs. Underwood was prescribed low-dose amitriptyline (Elavil®) when she first reported the zoster rash to her doctor, but it was discontinued owing to dry mouth, light-headedness, and sedation. She was later switched to desipramine (Norpramin®), which also caused intolerable sedation. At her current consultation, she was provided with an educational flyer (Box 2) and prescribed 300 mg of gabapentin (Neurontin®) daily, titrated to 1800 mg daily in divided doses. She was also prescribed a 5% lidocaine patch (Lidoderm®). Because of the area of her pain, she used two patches over her painful area, 12 hours on, then

Table 9
Targeted Treatment of Myofascial Pain

Nonmedication		Medication
• Restorative treatment	○ Physical therapy reconditioning and stretching exercises	○ Possibly trigger-point injections
• Preventive therapies	○ Physical therapy reconditioning and stretching exercises ○ Occupational therapy pacing and body mechanics	○ None
• Flare techniques	○ Physical therapy modalities ○ Stretching exercises ○ Trigger-point compression ○ Spray and stretch ○ Relaxation techniques	○ NSAIDs ○ Tramadol ○ Tizanidine ○ Trigger-point injections

NSAIDs, nonsteroidal anti-inflammatory drugs.

12 hours off. Her pain lessened, and she also felt protected from inadvertent touch when she wore the lidocaine patches. Mrs. Underwood was also recommended to complete BMD testing as part of her routine care, begin weight-bearing exercises, and add calcium and vitamin D supplements to her diet.

2.3. Myofascial Pain

The primary treatment of myofascial pain is physical therapy focusing on active stretching and range of motion exercises (Table 9). A home program of trigger-point compression therapy, stretching exercises, and postural correction effectively reduces myofascial thoracic pain *(34)*. After a therapist has helped identify trigger points and provided compression instruction, patients can apply pressure to trigger points before stretching by using a Thera Cane® (a J-shaped cane with six knobs placed around the cane; available at http://www.theracane.com/index.html). Pressure may also be applied by leaning against or lying on a tennis ball. Trigger-point compression must be coupled with active stretching exercises. Physical therapy may be enhanced by supplementing treatment with spray and stretch vasocoolant spray (Fluori-Methane®) applied to the painful area before stretching and trigger-point injections with 0.5 to 1% lidocaine or 0.25 to 0.5% bupivacaine. Trigger-point injections are made with a 22- to 25-gauge needle inserted about 1 cm from the trigger point, with injection of 0.1 to 0.2 mL of anesthetic. This process is repeated until a local twitch is no longer produced, muscle tightness is reduced, or 0.5 to 1 mL of anesthetic has been injected. Adding steroids to anesthetics does not improve pain relief duration. Acupuncture provides only temporary relief of myofascial thoracic pain (about 4–6 days relief *[53]*). Analgesics and muscle relaxants are minimally helpful for chronic myofascial pain. Analgesics may be used for occasional pain flares. One muscle relaxant, tizanidine (Zanaflex®), reduced pain by 58% and improved sleep by 69% when administered initially

---

Box 3
Educational Flyer for Myofascial Thorax Pain

What is myofascial pain?

Myofascial pain comes from the muscles (*myo*) and surrounding soft tissues (*fasciae*). Injury or overuse often results in painful muscle spasm that may last long after an injury or episode of muscle overuse. These muscles become short and tender to the touch. Pressing certain areas, called *trigger points*, may cause increased pain. Stretching the muscles may be initially painful, but continued gentle stretching usually eases the pain.

The muscles in your chest, around the shoulder blades, along the spine, and on the side of the ribs commonly develop myofascial pain. Trigger points in the muscles over your chest, around the shoulder blades, or on the side of the ribs often cause pain to travel into the arm. Trigger points in the muscles along the spine often send pain up into the shoulder blade or around to the front of the ribs.

How is myofascial pain treated?

Myofascial pain is most effectively treated with physical therapy and stretching exercises. Talk to your therapist about posture exercises and improving your work posture. Trigger points can be temporarily relieved with compression techniques or injections with steroid and numbing medicine. Spray and stretch using Fluori-Methane® is a numbing technique you and your therapist can use to help stretch muscles. Heat packs for 10 to 20 minutes may also be used before stretching exercises. Although most muscle relaxants are not helpful for myofascial pain, one called Zanaflex® (tizanidine) may help some patients. Learning psychological techniques to relax muscles and proper pacing of activities can also reduce myofascial pain.

Stretching exercises should be done twice daily and when pain flares up:

- Sit up straight on the edge of a chair in front of a desk. Hold the edge of the desk with both hands, with palms up and elbows bent to 90°. Gently lean backward, arching your upper back. Feel a stretch between your shoulder blades. Hold for 15 seconds. Repeat.
- Sit in a firm chair with your feet flat on the floor. Slowly bend forward until your head is resting on your knees and your hands are touching the floor by your feet. Hold for 15 seconds. Then sit up straight. Repeat.
- Stand in an open doorway with your right foot about 12 inches in front of you. Bend your right knee. Place your hands on the doorway at shoulder height. Slightly lean forward into the open doorway and feel the stretch across your chest. Hold for 10 seconds. Relax and repeat.

You should also use a firm, straight-backed chair at your desk. Adjust the chair height to avoid bending over to work. Putting a brick under your feet may also help your posture.

Where can I learn more about myofascial pain?

Good information about myofascial pain and its treatment can be found at these websites:

- http://my.webmd.com/content/article/100/105633.htm
- http://gasnet.med.yale.edu/local/pain/html/faq.html

as 2 mg at bedtime, and then increased as needed to a maximum of 12 mg daily in divided doses to patients with cervical myofascial pain *(36)*. Anecdotally, Zanaflex is also beneficial for myofascial thoracic pain. Mrs. Wilkins was provided with an educational flyer on myofascial pain (Box 3). A physical therapist treated her with spray and stretch using dichlorodifluoromethane–trichloromonofluoromethane (Fluori-Methane) followed by passive muscle stretching and instructions for active stretching exercises. She was advised to maintain a daily full-body stretching program to be performed twice daily in anticipation of hiking and camping outings. She was also recommended to complete BMD testing as part of her routine care and add calcium and vitamin D supplements to her diet.

3. SUMMARY

Each of these four women has multiple osteoporosis predictors, including age, female gender, menopausal status, and other risk factors. Every woman should be counseled about diet and exercise to achieve and maintain good bone health, and all should be screened with BMD after age 65. It is important to recognize, however, that osteoporosis is only one of many possible causes of thoracic pain. Thoracic pain will most commonly be caused by benign musculoskeletal conditions. Because of the vascular patterns around the thoracic spine, however, this region is a common area for metastatic disease, warranting a more in-depth evaluation for serious pathology than most cases of lower back pain.

REFERENCES

1. Wood KB, Garvey TA, Gundry C, Heithoff KB. Magnetic resonance imaging of the thoracic spine. Evaluation of asymptomatic individuals. J Bone Joint Surg Am 1995;77:1631–1638.
2. Delmas PD, van de Langerijt L, Watts NB, et al. Underdiagnosis of vertebral fractures is a worldwide problem: the IMPACT study. J Bone Miner Res 2005;20: 557–563.
3. Cuenod CA, Laredo JD, Chevret S, et al. Acute vertebral collapse due to osteoporosis or malignancy: appearance on unenhanced and gadolinium-enhanced MR images. Radiology 1996;199:541–549.
4. Tan DY, Tsou IY, Chee TS. Differentiation of malignant vertebral collapse from osteoporotic and other benign causes using magnetic resonance imaging. Ann Acad Med Singapore 2002;31:8–14.
5. Fu TS, Chen LH, Liao JC, et al. Magnetic resonance imaging characteristics of benign and malignant vertebral fractures. Chang Gung Med J 2004;27:808–815.
6. Kanis JA, Johnell O, Oden A, et al. Risk of hip fracture according to the World Health Organization criteria for osteopenia and osteoporosis. Bone 2000;27: 585–590.

7. Lindsay R, Pack S, Li Z. Longitudinal progression of fracture prevalence through a population of postmenopausal women with osteoporosis. Osteoporos Int 2005; 16:306–312.

8. Nevitt MC, Cummings SR, Stone KL, et al. Risk factors for a first-incident radiographic vertebral fracture in women > or = 65 years of age: the study of osteoporotic fractures. J Bone Miner Res 2005;20:131–140.

9. Barrett-Connor E, Siris ES, Wehren LE, et al. Osteoporosis and fracture risk in women of different ethnic groups. J Bone Miner Res 2005;20:185–194.

10. Edwards BJ, Iris M, Ferkel E, Feinglass J. Postmenopausal women with minimal trauma fractures are unapprised of the existence of low bone mass or osteoporosis. Maturitas 2006;53:260–266.

11. Simonelli C, Weiss TW, Morancey J, Swanson L, Chen Y. Prevalence of vitamin D inadequacy in a minimal trauma fracture population. Curr Med Res Opin 2005; 21:1069–1074.

12. Jung BF, Johnson RW, Griffin DR, Dworkin RH. Risk factors for postherpetic neuralgia in patients with herpes zoster. Neurology 2004;11:1545–1551.

13. Levack P, Graham J, Collie D, et al. Don't wait for a sensory level—listen to the symptoms: a prospective audit of the delays in diagnosis of malignant cord compression. Clin Oncol 2002;14:472–480.

14. Kanis JA, McCloskey EV, Powles T, et al. A high incidence of vertebral fracture in women with breast cancer. Br J Cancer 1999;79:1179–1181.

15. Lipton A. Management of bone metastases in breast cancer. Curr Treat Options Oncol 2005;6:161–171.

16. Pinski J, Dorff TB. Prostate cancer metastases to bone: pathophysiology, pain management, and the promise of targeted therapy. Eur J Cancer 2005;41:932–940.

17. Rosen LS, Gordon D, Kaminski M, et al. Long-term efficacy and safety of zoledronic acid compared with pamidronate disodium in the treatment of skeletal complications in patients with advanced multiple myeloma or breast carcinoma: a randomized, double-blind, multicenter, comparative trial. Cancer 2003;98: 1735–1744.

18. Brown JE, Neville-Webbe H, Coleman RE. The role of bisphosphonates in breast and prostate cancers. Endocr Relat Cancer 2004;11:207–224.

19. Vitamin D and calcium intakes from food or supplements and mammographic breast density. Cancer Epidemiol Biomarkers Pre 2005;14:1653–1659.

20. Gennari C. Calcium and vitamin D nutrition and bone disease of the elderly. Public Health Nutr 2001;4:547–559.

21. Chan K, Qin L, Lau M, et al. A randomized, prospective study of the effects of Tai Chi Chun exercise on bone mineral density in postmenopausal women. Arch Phys Med Rehabil 2004;85:717–722.

22. Snow CM, Shaw JM, Winters KM, Witzke KA. Long–term exercise using weighted vests prevents hip bone loss in postmenopausal women. J Gerontol A Biol Sci Med Sci 2000;55:M489–M491.

23. Lippuner K. Medical treatment of vertebral osteoporosis. Eur Spine J 2003;12 (Suppl 2):S132–S141.

24. Hodsman AB, Bauer CD, Dempster DW, et al. Parathyroid hormone and teriparatide for the treatment of osteoporosis: a review of the evidence and suggested guidelines for its use. Endocr Rev 2005;26:688–703.

25. Kanis JA, Barton IP, Johnell O. Risedronate decreases fracture risk in patients selected solely on the basis of prior vertebral fracture. Osteoporos Int 2005;16: 475–482.
26. Brecht JG, Kruse HP, Mohrke W, Oestreich A, Huppertz E. Health-economic comparison of three recommended drugs for the treatment of osteoporosis. Int J Clin Pharmacol Res 2004;24:1–10.
27. Reid IR, Brown JP, Burckhardt P, et al. Intravenous zoledronic acid in postmenopausal women with low bone mineral density. N Engl J Med 2002;346:653–661.
28. Alper BS, Lewis PR. Does treatment of acute herpes zoster prevent or shorten postherpetic neuralgia? J Fam Pract 2000;49:255–264.
29. Dworkin RH, Schmader KE. Treatment and prevention of postherpetic neuralgia. Clin Infect Dis 2003;36:877–882.
30. Bowsher D. The effects of pre–emptive treatment of postherpetic neuralgia with amitriptyline: a randomized, double–blind, placebo–controlled trial. J Pain Symptom Manage 1997;13:327–331.
31. Kuraishi Y, Takasaki I, Nojima H, Shiraki K, Takahata H. Effects of the suppression of acute herpetic pain by gabapentin and amitriptyline on the incidence of delayed postherpetic pain in mice. Life Sci 2004;74:2619–2626.
32. Herr H. Prognostic factors of postherpetic neuralgia. J Korean Med Sci 2002;17: 655–659.
33. Dubinsky RM, Kabbani H, El-Chami A, Boutwell C, Ali H. Practice parameter: treatment of postherpetic neuralgia. An evidence-based report of the Quality Standards Subcommitttee of the American Academy of Neurology. Neurology 2004; 63:959–965.
34. Hanten WP, Olson SL, Butts NL, Nowicki AL. Effectiveness of a home program of ischemic pressure followed by sustained stretch for treatment of myofascial trigger points. Phys Ther 2000;80:997–1003.
35. Kung YY, Chen FP, Chaung HL, et al. Evaluation of acupuncture effect to chronic myofascial pain syndrome in the cervical and upper back regions by the concept of Meridians. Acupunct Electrother Res 2002;26:195–202.
36. Malanga GA, Gwynn MW, Smith R, Miller D. Tizanidine is effective in the treatment of myofascial pain syndrome. Pain Physician 2002;5:422–432.

6

Pain in the Low Back

CHAPTER HIGHLIGHTS

- Low back pain is one of the top five diagnoses at physician office visits.
- Work duties and stress are significant risk factors for low back pain.
- Flexing the low back improves symptoms of lumbar stenosis, but aggravates radicular pain.
- Back extension improves radicular pain, but aggravates lumbar stenosis.

* * *

This afternoon, you have four new 50-year-old male patients, each with a chief complaint of a *pain in the low back* that started 5 weeks ago at work. Each patient was evaluated with a lumbar magnetic resonance imaging (MRI) scan and diagnosed with a bulging disc. Each patient was recommended to obtain a surgical consultation after securing a referral from his primary care doctor. Here are the stories each patient tells your nurse:

Patient 1: Mr. Darby is a pharmaceutical representative whose pain began while lifting boxes of drug samples at work. "My back's okay when I'm just sitting around, but when I try to walk, it really flares up. I just can't keep up with the young salesmen with this darn pain."

Patient 2: Mr. Eastgate is a hospital custodian whose pain began while throwing bags of laundry. "I haven't worked for weeks. I can tell my boss thinks I'm faking the pain to get compensation. I keep telling him I can't do anything at home, so how can I possibly come back to work?! Every time I try to do some work around the house, my back flares up. My wife just laughs at me, 'You look like an old woman with your hands on your hips.'"

Patient 3: Mr. Franklin is a carpenter. "I haven't been able to work since the pain got so bad. All the young guys started calling me 'grandpa.' This miserable pain keeps me from doing anything other than sitting in a chair. I can't even take the dog for a walk anymore. The only time my back doesn't bother me is when I'm helping my wife do grocery shopping."

From: *Current Clinical Practice: Headache and Chronic Pain Syndromes:*
The Case-Based Guide to Targeted Assessment and Treatment
By: D. A. Marcus © Humana Press, Totowa, NJ

Patient 4: Mr. Georges is an auto mechanic. "I'm so tired of having this pain. I've
            lost my motivation for doing anything. My boss told me to stop coming to
            the garage since I couldn't do any work without my pain flaring up. Now
            I just sit moping around the house, which just makes the pain worse."

1. EVALUATING LOW BACK PAIN

Low back pain is common. A survey of 2000 people in a general population
sample identified low back pain within the preceding 30 days in 23% between
16 and 45 years old and 43% over 45 years old *(1)*. Data from the National
Ambulatory Medical Care Survey ranked low back pain as the fifth leading
diagnosis for physician office visits, after hypertension, pregnancy, well-care
exams, and respiratory infections *(2)*. Low back pain was diagnosed in about
3% of all office visits.

The chief complaints and brief histories in these four patients are typical; however, none has provided enough information to formulate an educated diagnosis.
Although each patient has the same primary complaint, differences in history
and examination can provide ready clues to diagnostic possibilities (Table 1).
Although each patient produced an abnormal MRI, imaging studies of the spine
are notorious for producing false-positive reports. Screening MRIs in a general
population of 413 adults 40 years of age found bulging discs in 28% and pro-
truded or herniated discs in 25%, with nerve root impingement in 43% *(3)*.
Interestingly, reports of back pain were not correlated with any of these MRI-
identified abnormalities. The prevalence of MRI abnormalities in asymptomatic adults typically increases with age. Similarly, provocative discography
testing in patients with a previous history of back surgery does not discriminate between currently symptomatic and asymptomatic patients *(4,5)*. Extracting important features to distinguish among common disorders depends on a
targeted evaluation that focuses on high-yield questions and examination findings that help differentiate among the many possible causes of low back pain.

1.1. Developing a High-Yield Targeted Evaluation of Low Back Pain

Low back pain evaluations should be targeted to help confirm or refute likely
clinical diagnoses. The same evaluation principles apply to each patient regarding features in the history, physical examination findings, and the need to proceed with testing. Details of the targeted examination are outlined in Table 2.
Neurological examination of the lower extremities to identify motor and sensory changes, suggesting nerve root impingement or lumbar radiculopathy, is
detailed in Fig. 1 and Table 3. Nerve conduction study with electromyography
(NCS/EMG) and MRI testing are appropriate for patients with neurological deficits (e.g., radiculopathy or multiple lumbosacral root involvement with cauda
equine syndrome).

Table 1
Common Causes of Low Back Pain

Disease category	Specific diseases
• Musculoskeletal	○ Myofascial pain
	○ Osteoarthritis
	○ Osteoporosis with fractures
• Neurological	○ Radiculopathy
• Neoplastic	○ Focal or metastatic cancer
• Infectious	○ Vertebral osteomyelitis
	○ Epidural abscess
• Referred pain	○ Gastric disease (ulcers, tumors, inflammatory illness)
	○ Renal colic
	○ Abdominal aortic aneurysm
	○ Uterine disease (endometriosis, tumors)

Table 2
Keys to a Targeted Evaluation of Low Back Pain

• History	○ Clarify pain location—complete pain drawing
	○ Identify additional medical conditions
	○ Record pain precipitants, including relationship to walking (level or hills) and postural changes (back flexion or extension)
	○ Obtain complete review of systems
• Physical examination	○ Musculoskeletal exam:
	▪ ROM and tenderness
	○ Neurological exam:
	▪ Gait and extremity strength, reflexes, and sensation
	○ Abdominal exam
	○ Pelvic examination, as appropriate
• Testing	○ X-ray of the lumbosacral spine for mechanical signs
	○ NCS/EMG for peripheral neuropathy versus cervical radiculopathy
	○ MRI for lumbar radiculopathy or cauda equine syndrome

MRI, magnetic resonance imaging; NCS/EMG, nerve conduction study/electromyography; ROM, range of motion.

Table 3
Lower Extremity Evaluation for Lumbar Radiculopathy

	Lumbar radiculopathy			
	L3	L4	L5	S1
Motor loss	Knee extension	Knee extension	Foot dorsiflexion (heel walking)	Foot plantar flexion (toe walking)
Reflex loss	Knee reflex	Knee reflex	None	Ankle jerk
Sensory loss	Anterior medial thigh	Medial lower leg	Lateral lower leg and great toe	Lateral foot and sole
Usually affected disc space	L2–L3	L3–L4	L4–L5	L5–S1

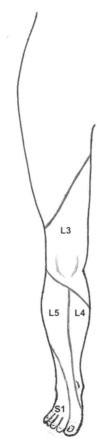

Fig. 1. Sensory distribution of lumbar nerve roots. Right lower extremity viewed from the anterior aspect. Skins areas served by specific lumbosacral nerve roots are marked. (Reprinted with permission from ref. *5a*.)

Work environment is a significant predictor for developing low back pain. Both physical demands (lifting, bending, twisting) and psychosocial factors (perceived stress, support, and job satisfaction) are important determinants of risk for low back pain. Each of our patients describes heavy work and work-related stressors. Premorbid patient characteristics predicting the development of chronic low back pain in patients with acute back pain include high psychological distress, poor self-rated health, low levels of physical activity, and dissatisfaction with employment *(6)*. Acute pain characteristics that predict chronic back pain include pain radiating to a lower extremity, widespread pain,

Table 4
Results of Targeted Evaluation for Patient 1:
Mr. Darby—50-Year-Old Salesman

Targeted assessment	Findings
History	○ Low back pain after lifting heavy sample boxes associated with burning in the lateral aspect of the left lower leg. Also, tingling in the left great toe. Leg pain increases every time his swings his leg forward to walk. Good general health.
Physical exam	
• Musculoskeletal	○ Vertebral muscle spasm and tenderness. Poor forward flexion with standing, which increases leg burning. Good extension.
• Neurological	○ Walks well on tip toes. Heel walking is poor on the left. Normal reflexes. Hypersensitivity to touch over anterior and lateral left lower leg. Numbness to pin in the left great toe.

and restricted range of motion in the back. Patients presenting with back pain should be queried about these features to help identify those patients at greater risk for more long-lasting back pain who, therefore, require more aggressive treatment of their acute pain episode. Smoking also increases the risk for developing chronic low back pain *(7)*. Risk is lower after patients have discontinued smoking.

1.2. Applying the Targeted Exam to Each Patient

Pain drawings are shown for each patient in Fig. 2. The results of the targeted evaluation are provided for each patient in Tables 4 to 7. In addition, each patient had a normal abdominal examination. Review the pain drawings, read each patient's findings, decide if additional testing is necessary, and formulate a likely diagnosis. Then read the following sections to compare your interpretations with the patients' diagnoses in the clinic.

1.2.1. Patient 1: Mr. Darby—50-Year-Old Pharmaceutical Salesman (Table 4)

Mr. Darby's pain drawing and physical examination reveal left lower extremity pain and neurological deficits, in addition to his back pain. His pain is also aggravated by lumbar flexion or swinging his leg forward to walk. NCS/EMG was performed to help confirm data on the clinical examination.

The NCS/EMG confirmed the clinical suspicion of a left L5 radiculopathy. Review of the previously obtained MRI revealed a left-sided disc at the L4–L5 interspace. Although a formal straight-leg raise test was not performed, the history of pain with raising the straight leg during walking and the inability to bend forward without pain when standing all describe the same maneuver.

A   Patient 1: Mr. Darby – 50-year-old salesman

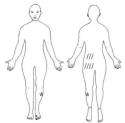

B   Patient 2: Mr. Eastgate – 50-year-old custodian

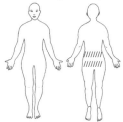

C   Patient 3: Mr. Franklin – 50-year-old carpenter

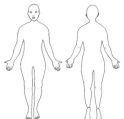

D   Patient 4: Mr. Georges – 50-year-old mechanic

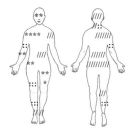

Fig. 2. Completed pain drawings for the four patients. (**A**) Patient 1: Mr. Darby—50-year-old salesman. (**B**) Patient 2: Mr. Eastgate—50-year-old custodian. (**C**) Patient 3: Mr. Franklin—50-year-old carpenter. (**D**) Patient 4: Mr. Georges—50-year-old mechanic.

Patients are instructed to shade all painful areas using the following key: //// = pain; :::::: = numbness; **** = burning or hypersensitivity

Table 5
Results of Targeted Evaluation for Patient 2:
Mr. Eastgate—50-Year-Old Custodian

Targeted assessment	Findings
History	○ Bilateral low back pain after 1 week with increased work duties when a co-worker was absent. No other pain areas. All movements aggravate his pain. Pain decreases with a heating pad. Typically inactive after work and on the weekends. ROS: Smokes two packs per day, peptic ulcer disease, depression.
Physical exam • Musculoskeletal	○ Moderately decreased active and passive ROM. Muscle tightness and tenderness bilaterally. Visible muscle spasm in the right low back. Palpating between the ribs and hip on the right causes a pain in the right buttock.
• Neurological	○ Normal screening exam

ROM, range of motion; ROS, review of systems.

Interestingly, the standard straight-leg raise test does not effectively discriminate pain caused by nerve root compression from other nondisc causes of radiating pain *(8)*. Formal straight-leg raise testing is best performed in the distracted patient when the patient is sitting at the bedside. The examiner can lift the foot to straighten the knee, creating a 90° straight-leg raise position. This is much more comfortable for patients than lifting the leg from a supine position. Patients often expect severe pain with a supine straight-leg raise and tend to tighten their lower back muscles, which further restricts movement, increases pain, and leads to an uninterpretable test.

1.2.2. Patient 2: Mr. Eastgate—50-Year-Old Custodian (Table 5)

Mr. Eastgate has multiple risk factors for low back pain (e.g., heavy work, low non-work activity level, depression, and smoking). These features suggest that he will likely need a more intensive treatment regimen to prevent the development of chronic low back pain. His examination and history reveal no neural or mechanical compromise. He does, however, have evidence of myofascial pain, with muscle spasm and an active trigger point in his quadratus lumborum muscle, rendering a diagnosis of quadratus lumborum myofascial pain syndrome.

Myofascial pain is characterized by tight and tender muscles with trigger points. A trigger point is a discrete area of tenderness within a muscle spasm. Pressing the trigger point may also cause pain to radiate in predictable patterns. The two most common lumbar myofascial syndromes are quadratus lumborum (low back and buttock pain) and piriformis (buttock and hip pain) syndromes.

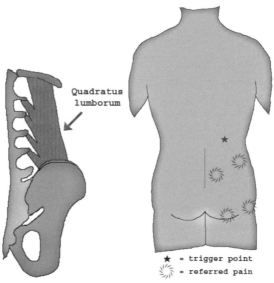

Fig. 3. Anatomy and referral patterns in quadratus lumborum syndrome. (Reprinted with permission ref. *5a*.)

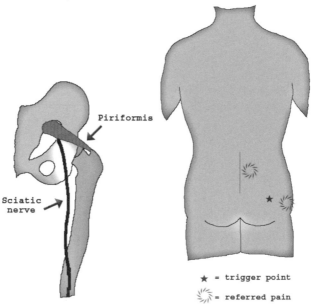

Fig. 4. Anatomy and referral patterns in piriformis syndrome. (Reprinted with permission from ref. *5a*.)

Table 6
Results of Targeted Evaluation for Patient 3:
Mr. Franklin—50-Year-Old Carpenter

Targeted assessment	Findings
History	○ Severe back and leg pain after walking about three blocks, which stops after sitting down. Walks better uphill, but only able to walk one block downhill. Good general health.
Physical exam	
• Musculoskeletal	○ Restricted back extension with good flexion. Minimal muscle tenderness.
• Neurological	○ Normal screening exam, including gait.

Muscle anatomy and typical location of trigger points and pain referral patterns in these syndromes are shown in Figs. 3 and 4. The quadratus lumborum muscles are the large posterior back muscles between the 12th rib and iliac crests that people rub when they say, "Oh, my aching back." The piriformis muscle connects the hip and femur. Piriformis tenderness can often be isolated during rectal or pelvic examinations.

1.2.3. Patient 3: Mr. Franklin—50-Year-Old Carpenter (Table 6)

Mr. Franklin's pain drawing is blank. He explains, "I don't have any pain unless I'm walking." Historical reports of pain aggravation with walking, development of a stoop ("walking like a grandpa" or improvement when stooping over a shopping cart), and better ability to walk uphill than downhill are all characteristic features of lumbar stenosis. History of relief with sitting is further suggestive of lumbar stenosis. Vascular claudication generally resolves with decreased activity (stopping walking) without any additional need to adjust posture, whereas forward flexion (readily achieved with sitting) is characteristically needed to reduce walking pain with lumbar stenosis. An X-ray of the lumbosacral spine with flexion and extension showed acceptable motion with no instability, and he was diagnosed with lumbar stenosis.

The diameter of the spinal canal decreases with back extension and increases with flexion. Like Mr. Franklin, lumbar stenosis patients are typically pain-free while sitting because this flexes the spine. Standing and walking reduce spine diameter. This diameter is further decreased when walking downhill because spine extension is needed to maintain appropriate center of gravity and balance with downhill walking. Stooping forward or sitting will relieve pain. Although spinal stenosis typically occurs in patients after age 65 years, a 5-year survey of all lumbar stenosis admissions found that 10% of patients were younger than 51 years old *(9)*. Physical examinations are typically normal in lumbar stenosis patients, with the exception of pain with extension, which

Table 7
Results of Targeted Evaluation for Patient 4:
Mr.Georges—50-Year-Old Mechanic

Targeted assessment	Findings
History	○ Pain affects low back everyday, with additional pain and numbness in many other body areas on different days.
	○ ROS: fatigue, poor sleep, bowel disturbance, anxiety, depression.
Physical exam	
• Musculoskeletal	○ Full ROM. Minimal tenderness to palpation over low back.
• Neurological	○ Normal screening exam.

ROM, range of motion; ROS, review of systems.

occurs in 69% of patients *(10)*. Because Mr. Franklin reports symptoms only with more prolonged walking, it is not surprising that his office examination, including hall walking, is normal.

1.2.4. Patient 4: Mr. Georges—50-Year-Old Mechanic (Table 7)

Mr. Georges' pain drawing and history reveal widespread pain complaints, as well as additional multisystem somatic and emotional complaints. Although his chief complaint was back pain, all of his symptoms must be considered when establishing a diagnosis. Because of his complaints, a fibromyalgia tenderpoint examination was performed, revealing 15 of 18 possible tenderpoints as positive. A complete discussion of Mr. Georges' diagnosis of fibromyalgia can be found in Chapter 10.

2. TREATING LOW BACK PAIN

Most episodes of acute low back pain resolve within several weeks. A total of 2487 patients with new low back pain were reassessed an average of 6 weeks after their initial consultation *(11)*. Low back pain was entirely resolved in 61%, improved in 33%, and unchanged or worsened in only 6%. Although the short-term prognosis of an episode of low back pain is good, low back pain tends to recur long-term, necessitating both treatment of the acute episode and strategies to prevent recurring pain. A 5-year prospective survey of 813 adults (ages 30–50 years) found that 40% with low back pain occurring for more than 30 days during the preceding year at the initial assessment similarly reported low back pain occurring for more than 30 days annually after 1 and 5 years *(12)*. Only 9% who experienced low back pain for more than 30 days during the first year were pain-free after 5 years. Likewise, a literature review of patients with low back pain noted that low back pain relapses after 1 year in 60%, with relapses of work absence in 33% *(13)*.

Bed rest is not necessary for managing low back pain. A randomized study compared 4 days of prescribed bed rest versus normal activities in patients with acute back pain or recurrent episodes of chronic low back pain *(14)*. Neither treatment resulted in significant differences in pain severity or disability, suggesting there is no advantage to excessive activity restrictions. In general, the most effective treatment for acute back pain is to maintain activities as tolerated, with no additional physical therapy or therapeutic exercise during the acute-pain phase *(15)*. When acute pain fails to diminish or chronic pain develops, this persistent pain is most effectively managed with stretches, strengthening, and mobility exercises *(15)*. Disability should also be specifically identified and addressed with physical and occupational therapy. Pooled data from two randomized treatment studies using workers with at least 4 to 8 weeks of work absence owing to low back pain showed an average superior reduction of work absence by 45 days over 12 months in patients treated with occupational therapy with work conditioning/hardening plus cognitive–behavioral instruction in comparison to treatment with routine conservative care *(16)*. Acupuncture, traction, and transcutaneous electrical nerve stimulation have not been shown to be consistently effective for acute or chronic low back pain *(15,17)*.

Disease-specific restorative treatments may be used to treat acute radiculopathy in Mr. Darby. Treating quadratus lumborum syndrome in Mr. Eastgate and lumbar stenosis in Mr. Franklin will necessitate long-term chronic pain management. Mr. Georges was provided with an educational flyer on fibromyalgia (available in Chapter 10), advised to begin a general body reconditioning and aerobic exercise program including walking, and prescribed Tofranil® (impiramine) to assist with sleep and mood disturbances. (A more complete discussion of fibromyalgia treatment may be found in Chapter 10.)

2.1. Lumbar Radiculopathy

Acute sciatica resolves within 4 weeks in up to 70% of patients, suggesting that initial treatment should be conservative and targeted to symptomatic improvement (*see* Table 8 and ref. *18*). Short-term treatment with systemic oral or locally infiltrated steroids, as well as oral nonsteroidal anti-inflammatory drugs (NSAIDs) often improves initial relief. A recent study demonstrated similar efficacy in patients treated with Voltaren® (diclofenac) or a Japanese serotonin-2A receptor antagonist, Anplag® (sarpogrelate) *(19)*. Periradicular infiltration of bupivacaine plus steroid results in short-term symptomatic improvement *(20)*. Patients with signs of multiple lumbosacral nerve compression (cauda equine syndrome) or persistent neurological loss (especially weakness) despite conservative management may require surgical decompression. Typically, lumbar decompression has lower efficacy when used for patients who report only pain or pain with numbness as the only neurological deficit. Although epidural injec-

Table 8
Targeted Treatment of Lumbar Radiculopathy

	Nonmedication	Medication
• Restorative treatment	○ Laminectomy, discectomy ○ Possibly physical therapy	○ Periradicular, epidural, or oral steroids
• Preventive therapies	○ Stretching and strengthening exercises ○ Pacing and body mechanics	○ Neuropathic medications
• Flare techniques	○ Physical therapy modalities ○ Stretching exercises ○ Relaxation techniques	○ NSAIDs ○ Muscle relaxants ○ Short-acting opioids for very severe pain unresponsive to other analgesics

NSAIDs, nonsteroidal anti-inflammatory drugs.

tions tend to be less effective than periradicular injections for lumbar radiculopathy, one study prospectively randomized patients with large lumbar disc herniations failing to improve after 6 weeks of conservative therapy to either epidural steroid injections or discectomy (21). Of the 169 patients enrolled in the study, symptoms improved during the initial conservative therapy for 69 (41%). The remaining 100 patients were equally randomized to epidural steroids or surgery. Pain reduction was greater with surgery during the first 2 years posttreatment, with pain similar between groups after 2 to 3 years. More patients treated with discectomy reported that their treatment was effective than with epidural steroids (about 95% versus 50%). Delaying surgery did not affect the outcome. The addition of postsurgical exercises further improves treatment outcome (22).

Patients with chronic radiculopathy or persistent sensory dysfunction after surgery may benefit from the addition of neuropathic medications. Antidepressants and some antiepileptic drugs (e.g., Neurotonin® [gabapentin] and Lamictal® [lamotrigine]) can significantly reduce painful hyperpathia and tingling, although numbness will persist (23,24).

Mr. Darby was provided with an educational flyer (Box 1) and prescribed Voltaren® (diclofenac) plus Zanaflex® (tizanidine) and advised to reduce activities to "as tolerated." Within 2 weeks, his leg symptoms had resolved and back pain was reduced by 50%. At that point, he was referred to physical therapy for modalities and a back-stabilizing exercise program.

2.2. Myofascial Low Back Pain

The primary treatment of myofascial pain is physical therapy focusing on active stretching and range-of-motion exercises (Table 9). Physical therapy may be enhanced by supplementing treatment with spray and stretch vasocoolant Fluori-Methane® spray applied to the painful area before stretching

---

Box 1
Educational Flyer for Lumbar Radiculopathy

What is a ruptured disc or pinched nerve?

Nerves can be pinched as they leave the spine to go into the leg. The area is called the *nerve root*. In Latin, *radicitus* means "by the roots." Therefore, when a nerve root is pinched in the low back (lumbar area), it is called a *lumbar radiculopathy*. When this happens, you may experience back pain, as well as pain, numbness, and/ or weakness in the leg.

The most common causes of pinched nerves are calcium deposits from arthritis or a herniated disc. The disc is a sponge-like cushion that acts like a shock absorber between the bones in the spine. Sometimes, this sponge can shift backward or to the side, causing the nerve to be pinched. With aging, this sponge dries out and causes the spaces between the bones to shrink, called *disc-space narrowing*. In addition, calcium deposits at these spaces and the nerves may get pinched, resulting in pain and numbness in the low back and leg. This leg pain is sometimes called *sciatica* because the sciatic nerve is commonly pinched in the lower back. Less commonly, people develop leg or foot weakness.

How is pinched nerve in the back treated?

Usually back pain from a pinched nerve or ruptured disc improves without surgery. Standard treatments include physical therapy, muscle relaxants, pain management therapies (such as stress management, relaxation, cognitive–behavioral therapies), and pain killers. Surgery is typically used when people have either: (1) leg or foot weakness, (2) problems with their bowels or bladder, or (3) no relief with nonsurgical treatments.

Under your doctor's supervision, exercises may also help reduce your pain:

• Lie flat on the floor on your belly. Bend your elbows and place your hands next to your head. Push your chest off of the floor, supporting the weight on your hands and elbows. Hold for 20 seconds. Relax and repeat.
• Lie flat on your belly with your hands folded behind your back. Lift your head and chest off of the floor. Hold 2 to 3 seconds. Relax and repeat.
• Lie on your back, knees bent, and the small of your back pressed into the floor. Keep your hands at your sides. Lift your head and shoulders up toward the ceiling. Hold 1 to 2 seconds. Relax and repeat.
• Lie on your back with one knee bent and the other leg straight. Press the small of your back into the floor. Lift the straight leg 4 inches off of the floor. Keeping this leg off of the floor, raise and lower it an additional 2 inches for 10 repetitions. Then switch sides and raise the other leg.

Where can I learn more about lumbar radiculopathy?

Good information about lumbar radiculopathy and its treatment can be found at these websites:

• http://www.mayoclinic.com/invoke.cfm?objectid=0000C8FB-D0CA-1B77-962480AEBC2F006D
• http://familydoctor.org/341.xml
• http://www.spine-health.com/

Table 9
Targeted Treatment of Myofascial Pain

	Nonmedication	Medication
• Restorative treatment	◦ Physical therapy reconditioning and stretching exercises	◦ Possibly trigger-point injections
• Preventive therapies	◦ Physical therapy reconditioning and stretching exercises ◦ Occupational therapy pacing and body mechanics	◦ Possibly botulinum toxin-A injections
• Flare techniques	◦ Physical therapy modalities ◦ Stretching exercises ◦ Trigger-point compression ◦ Spray and stretch ◦ Relaxation techniques	◦ NSAIDs ◦ Tramadol ◦ Tizanidine ◦ Trigger-point injection

NSAIDs, nonsteroidal anti-inflammatory drugs.

and trigger-point injections with 0.5 to 1% lidocaine or 0.25 to 0.5% bupivacaine. Injections should be made with a 22- to 25-gauge needle inserted about 1 cm distant from the trigger point and 0.1 to 0.2 mL of anesthetic should be injected. This process is repeated until a local twitch is no longer produced, muscle tightness is reduced, or 0.5 to 1 mL of anesthetic has been injected. The addition of steroid to anesthetic has not been shown to improve duration of pain relief. Patients failing to experience relief with physical therapy and other conservative measures may benefit from botulinum toxin-A injections. One open-label study of patients with refractory myofascial pain treated patients with 1-mL (10 U) botulinum toxin-A injections per site, for a total dosage of 50 U per injection session for patients injected in iliopsoas or quadratus lumborum muscles and 100 U in the piriformis *(25)*. Pain was modestly reduced (22%) after 3 months.

Analgesics and muscle relaxants are minimally helpful for chronic myofascial pain. Analgesics may be used for occasional pain flares. One muscle relaxant, Zanaflex® (tizanidine), has been shown to reduce pain by 58% and improve sleep by 69% when administered initially as 2 mg at bedtime and then increased as needed to a maximum of 12 mg daily in divided doses to patients with cervical myofascial pain *(26)*. Anecdotally, Zanaflex is also beneficial for myofascial lumbar pain.

Owing to multiple risk factors for chronic pain and the heavy nature of his required work duties, Mr. Eastgate began an aggressive initial pain management program. Mr. Eastgate was provided with an educational flyer (Box 2) and prescribed Zanaflex (tizanidine) and Ultram® (tramadol) rather than NSAIDs as a result of a history of peptic ulcer disease. He was also referred to physical therapy to begin a stretching and reconditioning program, with

---

Box 2
Educational Flyer for Myofascial Low Back Pain

What is myofascial low back pain?

   Myofascial pain describes pain coming from the muscles (*myo*) and surrounding soft tissues (*fasciae*). Injury or overuse often results in painful muscle spasm. In some cases, muscle spasm persists long after an injury or episode of muscle overuse. These muscles become short and tender to the touch. Pressing certain areas called *trigger points* may cause increased pain. Stretching the muscles may be initially painful, but continued stretching usually eases the pain.

   The two most common myofascial low back pains are quadratus lumborum and piriformis syndromes. The *quadratus lumborum* is a large rectangular muscle that attaches on top to the 12th rib, on the side to the spine, and on the bottom to the hip bone. This muscle stabilizes the back and allows you to bend to the side. If you put your hands on your hips, your thumbs will be in the middle of the quadratus lumborum muscles. Muscle pain involving the quadratus lumborum muscle is one of the most common causes of low back pain. It can also cause pain to go into the hip and buttock. The *piriformis* muscle is a long, thin muscle that connects the hip to the thigh bone in your hip socket. This muscle stabilizes and rotates the hip. Piriformis muscle pain causes pain in the hip and buttock, and sometimes the leg.

How is myofascial pain treated?

   Myofascial pain is most effectively treated with physical therapy and stretching exercises. Some doctors will temporarily ease your pain with an injection of steroid and numbing medicine into the muscle, called a *trigger-point injection*. Although most muscle relaxants are not helpful for myofascial pain, one called Zanaflex® (tizanidine) may help some patients. Learning psychological techniques to relax muscles and proper pacing of activities can also reduce myofascial pain.

   Stretching exercises should be done twice daily and may also be done when pain flares during the day. Many stretches can be done while sitting at your desk in the office:

- A simple way to stretch the quadratus lumborum muscle is to sit in a stiff chair and raise your arms overhead. Keeping your buttocks firmly on the chair, lean to the side away from the painful muscle. While leaning to the side, tip forward slightly. You should feel a gentle stretch in the quadratus lumborum muscle. Hold for 10 to 20 seconds; then repeat on the other side.
- To stretch your left piriformis muscle, sit in a stiff chair. Cross your left leg over the right. Use your hands to pull the bent left knee up and toward your chest. Turn your chest to face the left knee. You should feel a gentle stretch of the piriformis muscle in your left buttock. Hold for 10 to 20 seconds; then repeat on the right side.

Where can I learn more about myofascial pain?

   Good information about myofascial pain and its treatment can be found at these websites:

- http://my.webmd.com/content/article/100/105633.htm
- http://gasnet.med.yale.edu/local/pain/html/faq.html

Table 10
Targeted Treatment of Lumbar Stenosis

	Nonmedication	Medication
• Restorative treatment	∘ Decompressive surgery	∘ Epidural steroid injections
• Preventive therapies	∘ Postural correction	∘ None
	∘ Extension exercises	
• Flare techniques	∘ Postural correction	∘ NSAIDs
	∘ Extension exercises	∘ Epidural or oral steroids

NSAIDs, nonsteroidal anti-inflammatory drugs.

instructions to perform stretching exercises twice daily after applying heat to the low back for 20 minutes. In addition, he worked with an occupational therapist who reviewed his work duties and instructed him in better body mechanics and pacing techniques. The occupational therapist also provided a gradual re-entry schedule for work so that he was back to full-time duties within 2 weeks.

2.3. Lumbar Stenosis

Lumbar stenosis is treated with postural correction and strengthening exercises to improve spine flexion and reduce extension (Table 10). Epidural steroids are also at least temporarily helpful for most patients. Pain relief usually lasts 2 to 3 months, although relief may extend up to 1 year in some patients *(10)*. A review of 140 patients with lumbar stenosis who were treated with epidural steroid injections showed pain relief lasting less than 2 months in 39% and more than 2 months in 32% *(27)*. Patients with moderate to severe symptoms are typically managed surgically. Surgical decompression of lumbar stenosis is safe with good efficacy, even in patients 75 years of age or older *(28)*. In uncontrolled studies, short-term improvement is typically superior with surgical versus conservative treatment, although this difference lessens during long-term follow-up *(29)*. A prospective study followed 100 consecutive patients with lumbar stenosis for 10 years *(30)*. Those with initial severe symptoms ($n = 19$) were operated, whereas those with moderate symptoms were treated conservatively ($n = 50$). The remaining patients with moderate-to-severe pain were randomized to initial treatment with conservative therapy ($n = 18$) or surgery ($n = 13$). A good result was reported after 6 months, 1 year, and 4 years, respectively, by 79, 89, and 84% selected for surgery; 70, 64, and 57% for selected conservative treatment; 92, 69, and 92% randomly assigned to surgery; and 39, 33, and 47% randomly assigned to conservative treatment. Outcome was stable for the remaining 6 years of follow-up. Of those initially treated with conservative treatment, 29% were later operated on. Importantly, although patients fared better after surgery than conservative treatment alone, delaying surgery did not result in an inferior outcome compared with patients initially treated surgically. This study supports initial treatment of mild-to-moderate symptoms with conservative treatment before considering surgery.

Mr. Franklin was provided with an educational flyer (Box 3). Because his symptoms were fairly new in onset, he was treated with three epidural steroid injections each administered 2 weeks apart, and physical therapy to improve spine stability and posture. This resulted in good pain relief. At 6 months follow-up, he reported continued good pain relief unless he walked on steep hills or worked overhead, causing his back to extend backward.

3. SUMMARY

Although imaging studies of the lumbar spine typically show disc-space narrowing and bulging or herniated discs, lumbar disc disease is not the only, or even the most common, cause of persistent low back pain. A high-yield, targeted history and examination can help distinguish among the common causes of low back pain. Attention to patient posture and associated symptoms assists in correctly identifying whether an abnormal imaging study is likely to be related to a particular low back pain complaint.

REFERENCES

1. Stranjalis G, Tsamandouraki K, Sakas DE, Alamanos Y. Low back pain in a representative sample of Greek population. Analysis according to personal and socioeconomic characteristics. Spine 2004;29:1355–1362.
2. Hart LG, Deyo RA, Cherkin DC. Physician office visits for low back pain. Frequency, clinical evaluation, and treatment patterns from a U.S. national survey. Spine 1995;20:11–19.
3. Kjaer P, Leboeuf-Yde C, Korsholm L, Sorensen JS, Bendix T. Magnetic resonance imaging and low back pain in adults: a diagnostic imaging study of 40-year-old men and women. Spine 2005;30:1173–1180.
4. Carragee EJ, Chen Y, Tanner CM, Truong T, Lau E, Brito JL. Provocative discography in patients after limited lumbar discectomy: a controlled, randomized study of pain response in symptomatic and asymptomatic subjects. Spine 2000; 25:3065–3071.
5. Carragee EJ, Paraagioudakis SJ, Khurana S. 2000 Volvo Award winner in clinical studies: lumbar high-intensity zone and discography in subjects without low back problems. Spine 2000;25:2987–2992.
5a. Marcus DA. Chronic Pain: A Primary Care Guide to Practical Management. Totowa, NJ: Humana Press, 2005.
6. Thomas E, Silman AJ, Croft PR, et al. Predicting who develops chronic low back pain in primary care: a prospective study. BMJ 1999;318:1662–1667.

Box 3
Educational Flyer for Lumbar Stenosis

What is lumbar stenosis?

Your spine is made up of a column of bones, or *vertebrae*, that form a protective ring or canal around the nerves in your back. When you bend forward or backward, each individual bone moves a little differently to allow you to bend, twist, and turn (in Latin, *verto* means "to turn"). The canal space inside of the ring will be the greatest when all of the rings line up on top of each other. Because your spine is naturally curved, the holes inside the rings of the spine bones line up the best when you stoop forward. The space gets slightly smaller when you stand up straight, and is the smallest when you tilt backward. In most people, the size of the space is big enough for the nerves even when you bend backward. Some people, however, have a small space that causes the nerves to be pinched when they stand up straight or bend backward. This space can be small at birth or get smaller because of arthritis or injury. *Lumbar stenosis* or *spinal stenosis* is a narrowing (stenosis) of the space within your low back (lumbar region).

People with lumbar stenosis usually feel better when their spine is straight (such as with sitting) or bent forward. When the spine curves backward (which occurs normally with standing and walking) or you bend backward (which occurs when walking downhill), you will have back pain that often goes into the legs or is associated with leg numbness. You will probably notice your pain gets better once you sit down or stoop forward. That is because these postures help align the bones in the spine to open the space for the nerves.

How is lumbar stenosis treated?

Treatment usually consists of posture correction, epidural steroid injections, and, in many cases, surgery. Physical therapy exercises can help improve your posture and strengthen your abdominal muscles to reduce the backward curve in your spine. You will also want to avoid bending backward. When nerves become irritated, tissues may swell. This swelling will also reduce the space available for nerves. Nonsteroidal anti-inflammatory medications (such as Motrin® [ibuprofen]) and steroids help to temporarily reduce inflammation or swelling. Your doctor may inject a steroid into the space around your spine (epidural space). These injections will usually need to be repeated. When back and leg pain is severe or restricts your daily activities, your doctor may suggest surgery to remove some of the bone in your back to increase the space for the nerves. This surgery is called a *laminectomy* because the small parts of the spine (the laminae) are removed. The Latin word *laminae* means "plates" and the Greek work *ektome* means "remove." So a laminectomy is the removal of bony plates in the spine.

Where can I learn more about lumbar stenosis?

Good information about lumbar stenosis and its treatment can be found at these websites:

• http://familydoctor.org/256.xml
• http://www.neurosurgerytoday.org/what/patient_e/lumbar.asp
• www.back.com/causes-mechanical-stenosis.html

7. Andersson H, Ejlertsson G, Leden I. Widespread musculoskeletal chronic pain associated with smoking. An epidemiological study in a general rural population. Scand J Rehabil Med 1998;30:185–191.
8. Vroomen PJ, de Krom MM, Wilmink JT, Kester AM, Knottnerus JA. Diagnostic value of history and physical examination in patients suspected of lumbosacral nerve root compression. J Neurol Neurosurg Psychiatry 2002;72:630–634.
9. LaBan MM, Imas A. "Young" lumbar spinal stenotic: review of 268 patients younger than 51 years. Am J Phys Med Rehabil 2003;82:69–71.
10. Radu AS, Menkes CJ. Update on lumbar spinal stenosis. Retrospective study of 62 patients and review of the literature. Rev Rhum Engl Ed 1998;65:337–345.
11. Valat J, Goupille P, Rozenberg S, Urbinelle R, Allaert F. Acute low back pain: predictive index of chronicity from a cohort of 2487 subjects. Joint Bone Spine 2000;67:456–461.
12. Hestbaek L, Leboeuf-Yde C, Engberg M, et al. The course of low back pain in a general population. Results from a 5-year prospective study. J Manipulative Physiol Ther 2003;26:213–219.
13. Hestbaek L, Leboeuf-Yde C, Manniche C. Low back pain: what is the long-term course? A review of studies of general patient populations. Eur Spine J 2003;12: 149–165.
14. Rozenberg S, Delval C, Rezvani Y, et al. Bed rest of normal activity for patients with acute low back pain. A randomized controlled trial. Spine 2002;27:1487–1493.
15. Harris GR, Susman JL. Managing musculoskeletal complaints with rehabilitation therapy: summary of the Philadelphia Panel evidence-based clinical practice guidelines on musculoskeletal rehabilitation interventions. J Fam Pract 2002;51: 1042–1046.
16. Schonstein E, Kenny D, Keating J, Koes B. Physical conditioning programs for workers with back and neck pain: a Cochrane systemic review. Spine 2003;28: E391–E395.
17. van Tulder MW, Cherkin DC, Berman B, Lao L, Koes BW. The effectiveness of acupuncture in the management of acute and chronic low back pain. A systematic review within the framework of the Cochrane Collaboration Back Review group. Spine 1999;24:1113–1123.
18. Weber H, Holme I, Amlie E. The natural course of acute sciatica with nerve root symptoms in a double-blind placebo-controlled trial evaluating the effect of piroxicam. Spine 1993;18:1433–1438.
19. Kanayama M, Hashimoto T, Shigenobu K, Oha F, Yamane S. New treatment of lumbar disc herniation involving 5-hydroxytryptamine 2A receptor inhibitor: a randomized controlled trial. J Neurosurg Spine 2005;2:441–446.
20. Karppinen J, Malmivaara A, Kurunlahti M, et al. Periradicular infiltration for sciatica: a randomized controlled trial. Spine 2001;26:1059–1067.
21. Buttermann GR. Treatment of lumbar disc herniation: epidural steroid injection compared with discectomy. A prospective, randomized study. J Bone Joint Surg Am 2004;86-A:670–679.
22. Filiz M, Cakmak A, Ozcan E. The effectiveness of exercise programmes after lumbar disc surgery: a randomized controlled study. Clin Rehabil 2005;19:4–11.

23. Eisenberg E, Damunni G, Hoffer E, Baum Y, Krivoy N. Lamotrigine for intractable sciatica: correlation between dose, plasma concentration and analgesia. Eur J Pain 2003;7:485–491.
24. Baron R, Binder A. How neuropathic is sciatica? The mixed pain concept. Orthopade 2004;33:568–575.
25. De Andrés J, Cerda-Olmedo G, Valía JC, et al. Use of botulinum toxin in the treatment of chronic myofascial pain. Clin J Pain 2003;19:269–275.
26. Malanga GA, Gwynn MW, Smith R, Miller D. Tizanidine is effective in the treatment of myofascial pain syndrome. Pain Physician 2002;5:422–432.
27. Delport EG, Cucuzzella AR, Marley JK, Pruitt CM, Fisher JR. Treatment of lumbar spinal stenosis with epidural steroid injections: a retrospective outcome study. Arch Phys Med Rehabil 2004;85:479–484.
28. Fredman B, Arinzon Z, Zohar E, et al. Observations on the safety and efficacy of surgical decompression for lumbar spinal stenosis in geriatric patients. Eur Spine 2002;11:571–574.
29. Atlas SJ, Keller RB, Wu YA, Deyo RA, Singer DE. Long-term outcomes of surgical and nonsurgical management of lumbar spinal stenosis: 8 to 10 year results from the Maine lumbar spine study. Spine 2005;30:936–943.
30. Amundsen T, Weber H, Nordal HJ, et al. Lumbar spinal stenosis: conservative or surgical management?: a prospective 10-year study. Spine 2000;25:1424–1435.

7

Pain in the Hand

CHAPTER HIGHLIGHTS

- Compressive neuropathies occur more frequently during pregnancy.
- Physical and occupational therapists offer important rehabilitative treatment for patients with hand pain.
- Most common hand pain syndromes can be effectively treated without surgery.

* * *

This afternoon, you have three new patients, each of whom complains of *a pain in the hand*. They are all here for an initial consultation. Here are the stories each patient tells your nurse:

Patient 1: Mrs. Miller is a 33-year-old mother of two: "Ever since I had my new baby, all I seem to do is complain. It hurts to take care of the kids. It hurts to prepare meals. And forget about gardening, which I used to love. My family thinks it must be postpartum depression."

Patient 2: Mrs. Nealy is a 35-year-old primigravida: "I used to laugh at my friends who complained about stomach upset, swelling, and back pain with pregnancy. Since I've been pregnant, it seems like everything's bothering me, too. Ever since my seventh month, my hands are just unbearable. They keep me from working during the day and sleeping at night."

Patient 3: Miss Olds is a 47-year-old English teacher: "My hand has been killing me for the last 6 months. The pain has even spread to my arm now. Everything seems to set it off. I just want to sit behind my desk and hide."

1. EVALUATING HAND PAIN

A recent survey of 5752 patients registered with a primary care practitioner identified hand pain in 7% of men and women between the ages of 16 and 44 and 13% of men and 20% of women 45 years of age or older *(1)*. A similar survey of 6038 adult primary care patients (ages 25–64 years) reported a spe-

From: *Current Clinical Practice: Headache and Chronic Pain Syndromes:*
The Case-Based Guide to Targeted Assessment and Treatment
By: D. A. Marcus © Humana Press, Totowa, NJ

Table 1
Common Causes of Hand Pain

Disease category	Specific diseases
• Musculoskeletal	∘ Traumatic (e.g., sprain or fracture)
	∘ Arthritic (e.g., rheumatoid arthritis)
	∘ Compressive tenosynovitis (e.g., De Quervain's syndrome)
	∘ Ganglion cyst
• Neuropathic	∘ Compressive neuropathy (e.g., carpal tunnel syndrome)
	∘ Complex regional pain syndrome
• Vascular	∘ Raynaud's syndrome

cific hand and/or wrist pain syndrome (De Quervain's wrist tenosynovitis or carpal tunnel syndrome) in about 3% of patients, with nonspecific hand and/or wrist pain in about 10% *(2)*. Hand pain can significantly impair both work and leisure activities.

Although the chief complaints and brief histories of these three patients are typical, none has provided enough information to formulate an educated diagnosis. Each patient has the same primary complaint; however, differences in history and examination can provide ready clues to diagnostic possibilities (Table 1). Extracting important features to distinguish among common disorders depends on a targeted evaluation that focuses on high-yield questions and examination findings that help distinguish among the many possible causes of hand pain.

1.1. Developing a High-Yield Targeted Evaluation of Hand Pain

Evaluations of patients with hand pain should be targeted to specific likely clinical scenarios to help confirm or refute clinical diagnoses. The same evaluation principles apply to each patient regarding features in the history, physical examination findings, and the need to proceed with testing. Details of the targeted examination are outlined in Table 2. The following special tests to identify common entrapment syndromes can be readily performed at the bedside:

1. Finkelstein's test for stenosing tenosynovitis of the first dorsal compartment (De Quervain's syndrome; Fig. 1).
2. Phalen's test (in which patients are asked to flex the wrist for 1 minute) and percussion of the carpal tunnel for median nerve entrapment in the wrist.
3. Palpation of the ulnar nerve at the elbow for ulnar nerve entrapment.

The development of increased pain or hand paresthesias with these maneuvers helps to confirm a clinical suspicion of common entrapment syndromes. Patients with limited hand motion, joint deformities, crepitus, or point tenderness generally require an imaging study to rule out joint disease or fracture.

Table 2
Keys to a Targeted Evaluation of Hand Pain

• History	○ Clarify pain location—complete pain drawing
	○ Record pain precipitants, such as injury or trauma
	○ Note any neurological deficits or functional loss
	○ Note any other limb abnormalities
	(sensitivity to touch, temperature, and growth of hair and nails)
	○ Identify aggravating factors
	○ Identify additional medical conditions
	○ Obtain complete review of systems
• Physical examination	○ Musculoskeletal exam:
	▪ joint inspection for deformities, neck and upper extremity ROM and tenderness, and Finkelstein's test for thumb pain.
	○ Neurological exam:
	▪ Gait, extremity strength, reflexes and sensation. Phalen's test, percussion of the median nerve at the wrist, and firm palpation of the ulnar nerve at the elbow.
• Testing	▪ X-ray of the wrist and hand when trauma has occurred or mechanical signs are present.
	○ NCS/EMG for peripheral neuropathy versus cervical radiculopathy

NCS/EMG, nerve conduction studies/electromyography; ROM, range of motion.

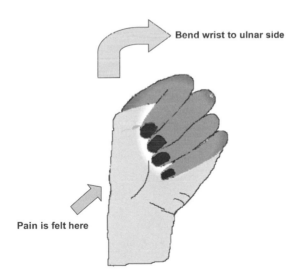

Fig. 1. Finkelstein's test for De Quervain's tenosynovitis. Finkelstein's test is performed by asking the patient to make a fist, with the thumb placed under the fingers. The examiner then bends the wrist away from the thumb toward the ulnar side. A positive test occurs when the patient reports pain in the wrist at the base of the thumb.

A   Patient 1: Mrs. Miller – 33-year-old mother

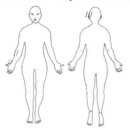

B   Patient 2: Mrs. Nealy – 35-year-old pregnant woman

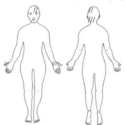

C   Patient 3: Ms. Olds – 47-year-old teacher

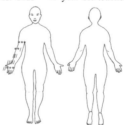

Fig. 2. Completed pain drawings for the three patients. (**A**) Patient 1: Mrs. Miller—33-year-old mother. (**B**) Patient 2: Mrs. Nealy—35-year-old pregnant woman. (**C**) Patient 3: Ms. Olds—47-year-old teacher.

Patients are instructed to shade all painful areas using the following key: //// = pain; :::::: = numbness; **** = burning or hypersensitivity.

1.2. Applying the Targeted Exam to Each Patient

Pain drawings for each patient are shown in Fig. 2. The results of the targeted evaluation for each patient are provided in Tables 3 to 5. Review the pain drawings, read each patient's findings, decide if additional testing is necessary, and formulate a likely diagnosis. Then read the following sections to compare your interpretations with the patients' diagnoses in the clinic.

Table 3
Results of Targeted Evaluation for Patient 1:
Mrs. Miller—33-Year-Old Mother

Targeted assessment	Findings
• History	○ No preceding injury or trauma
	○ No numbness. Hand is weak.
	○ Pain is aggravated by lifting and breastfeeding her new baby, opening jars, picking up her child's small toys. "If this pain doesn't go away soon, I'm switching to bottle feeding."
	○ Good general health. She is using no medications other than prenatal vitamins because she is still nursing her baby.
	○ Normal ROS
Physical exam	
• Musculoskeletal	○ No tenderness and normal ROM of her neck and proximal upper extremity. Tenderness over base of right thumb. Full ROM in hand and wrist. No joint swelling or crepitus. Pain is aggravated by Finkelstein's test.
• Neurological	○ Gait testing was normal. Good sensation, strength, and reflexes in the arms. Negative Phalen's test. Mild local tenderness with percussion of the median nerve. The ulnar nerve is tender to palpation at the elbow.

ROM, range of motion; ROS, review of systems.

1.2.1. *Patient 1: Mrs. Miller—33-Year-Old Mother* (Table 3)

Mrs. Miller's primary pain is in the right thumb, with some pain going into the forearm. She also has infrequent, mild migraine headaches. There is no report of paresthesia or allodynia, and no sensory disturbance noted on physical examination. Although she reports hand weakness, testing shows normal strength, suggesting her perceived weakness reflects limitations resulting from pain. There is tenderness over the base of the thumb, but she has full range of motion and no joint crepitus. Finkelstein's test is positive, with negative Phalen's test. Percussion or palpation of the median and ulnar nerves produces local discomfort with no radiation. Lack of mechanical signs and neurological symptoms preclude testing with X-rays or nerve conduction studies (NCSs). Mrs. Miller is diagnosed with stenosing tenosynovitis, or De Quervain's syndrome.

De Quervain's tenosynovitis is a common painful inflammatory condition of the thumb. The tendons for the abductor pollicis longus and extensor pollicis brevis travel into the thumb through a small compartment in the wrist. When the thumb is extended, these tendons can be seen at the base of the thumb, where they form the radial border of the anatomic snuff box. Inflammation of the synovial lining of this tunnel can impair the ability of these tendons to slide

Table 4
Results of Targeted Evaluation for Patient 2:
Mrs. Nealy—35-Year -Old Pregnant Woman

Targeted assessment	Findings
History	○ No preceding injury or trauma
	○ No numbness, but she gets shooting pains and tingling into her right thumb and index finger when she types at work and in both hands in the middle of the night.
	○ History of migraine, which resolved during her second trimester. She is taking only prenatal vitamins and acetaminophen.
	○ ROS remarkable for panic disorder (currently controlled)
Physical exam	
• Musculoskeletal	○ Full ROM of her neck and upper extremities. Finkelstein's maneuver minimally aggravates her pain.
• Neurological	○ Normal gait. Good strength, sensation, and reflexes in her upper and forearms. Thumb opposition is weak in her right hand. Allodynia over her right thenar eminence and the tip of her right index finger. Phalen's test aggravates pain in both hands. Percussion of the wrist is not painful and palpation of the ulnar nerve is minimally uncomfortable.

ROM, range of motion; ROS, review of systems.

smoothly, resulting in pain. Inflammation may occur as a result of trauma or repetitive overuse injury. Patients with diabetes, thyroid disease, and rheumatoid arthritis are also at high risk for developing De Quervain's syndrome. The pain is typically aggravated by grasping, twisting, or pinching with the hand and thumb, explaining Mrs. Miller's discomfort with lifting, opening jars, and picking up small toys. A report of De Quervain's syndrome during pregnancy or postpartum noted frequent worsening after delivery, with the most severe symptoms occurring while breastfeeding *(3)*.

1.2.2. Patient 2:
Mrs. Nealy—35-Year-Old in Third Trimester of Pregnancy (Table 4)

Mrs. Nealy's pain drawing shows her chief complaint of pain in both hands and intermittent migraine, which has improved during her pregnancy. Musculoskeletal testing is normal. Sensory disturbance and motor loss are noted in her dominant right hand. Phalen's test is positive bilaterally, with no tenderness to percussion of the carpal tunnel. No additional testing is ordered, and she is diagnosed with compression of the median nerve at the wrist, or carpal tunnel syndrome. NCSs may be used to confirm a clinical diagnosis of carpal tunnel syndrome, especially in patients failing to respond to conservative measures or who are being considered for injections or surgical decompression. In general, median nerve conduction across the wrist is delayed in pregnant

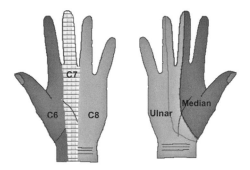

Fig. 3. Comparison of sensory loss from radiculopathy versus peripheral.

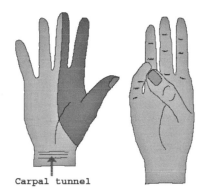

Fig. 4. Carpal tunnel syndrome.

women, although comparing delays in median and ulnar nerve conduction in pregnant women can effectively discriminate symptomatic from asymptomatic delays *(4)*.

The median nerve supplies sensation to the lateral aspect of the hand, over the thumb and first two fingers (Fig. 3). This nerve also supplies motor function to the thenar eminence, allowing opposition of the thumb (Fig. 4). Pain and dysesthesia are typically aggravated by compressing or stretching the wrist and sleeping, possibly owing to the combination of wrist hyperextension or flexion with sleep and increased hand swelling with expected fluid redistribution while lying down. Carpal tunnel symptoms may be aggravated or reproduced with the Phalen's test (in which patients are asked to flex the wrist for 1 minute) and percussion of the carpal tunnel. Production of tingling in the thumb, index, and middle fingers with percussion is a positive Tinel's sign. Phalen and wrist percussion testing were evaluated in 112 patients with clinical carpal tunnel syndrome confirmed by NCSs and 50 pain-free controls *(5)*. The sensitivity and specificity, respectively, were 85 and 89% for Phalen's test and 67 and 68% for Tinel's sign. Interestingly, both of these tests were negative in 17 patients with confirmed carpal tunnel syndrome (15%). A positive Phalen's test is also associated with increased carpal tunnel syndrome severity, suggesting that follow-up Phalen's testing may help to identify treatment effectiveness *(6)*.

A longitudinal study following workers for an average of 5.4 years identified pre-existing hand symptoms, obesity, diabetes, and perceived stress as risk factors for developing carpal tunnel symptoms *(7)*. Median nerve compression at the wrist under the carpal tunnel may also occur during pregnancy. A prospective evaluation of 100 pregnant women with clinical assessment and NCSs identified carpal tunnel syndrome in 17% (25% of women assessed during the first trimester, 11% during the second trimester, and 19% during the third trimester *[8]*). Symptoms were bilateral in 24% and severe in 18%. A survey of obstetrical patients in their eight and ninth months of pregnancy identified pre-existing carpal tunnel symptoms in 12% and pregnancy-related carpal tunnel in 50% *(9)*. Paresthesias were reported in both hands in 41% of the patients in this survey. Carpal tunnel symptoms during pregnancy are different from nonpregnancy carpal tunnel syndrome because pregnant women often complain of bilateral sensory symptoms and motor loss *(10)*.

1.2.3. Patient 3: Ms. Olds—47-Year-Old Teacher (Table 5)

Ms. Olds' pain began about 2 months after a wrist sprain that was treated with splinting. X-rays at the time of her injury were reviewed and showed no fracture or other abnormality. Her examination is extremely limited because of her reports of pain. The examiner asked Ms. Olds to move through her range as much as possible, and she demonstrated fair range of motion throughout the right upper extremity. Passive range of motion could not be performed. Ms. Olds' history and posture are consistent with the diagnosis of complex regional pain syndrome (CRPS). There are no specific tests to confirm the diagnosis of CRPS.

Patients with CRPS characteristically guard their painful extremity, often splinting the arm and trying to limit any sensory stimulation. Pain reports typically seem excessively high for the provocative injury *(11)*. Patients typically report changes in temperature of the painful limb, as well as intermittent redness and swelling. These findings may or may not be evident at the time of evaluation, as they are generally transient. Interestingly, patient's subjective reports of CRPS changes (allodynia, edema, sweating/color/temperature abnormality) have greater diagnostic sensitivity and specificity than

Table 5
Results of Targeted Evaluation for Patient 3:
Mrs. Olds—47-Year-Old Teacher

Targeted assessment	Findings
History	○ Fell on the ice 7 months ago, and sprained her right wrist. She wore a short splint for 2 months, but the pain seemed to just get worse. ○ She has no numbness and says she cannot move the right hand at all. ○ Pain is aggravated by touching the hand or arm or when someone bumps into her. She cannot stand to get the hand cold, so she tends to wear a shawl over the arm. ○ She often feels her hand is ice cold, but the temperature always seems the same as the left hand when she sees the doctor. She also complains that her hand often swells and turns pink. There are no changes in her arm hair or nails, but she stopped cutting the nails on her right hand because it hurt too much. ○ Good general health. She has never been prescribed medications for her pain, but has used a variety of pain pills left over from previous dental procedures. These have been minimally helpful. ○ ROS unremarkable
Physical exam • Musculoskeletal	○ Patient refuses all testing of the right upper extremity by the examiner, although she can demonstrate fair active motion. ROM of the neck and left upper extremity are normal. No swelling is noted.
• Neurological	○ Patient refuses all testing of the right upper extremity. Neurological examination of the left upper extremity is normal. Gait testing is normal, except that she walks with her right upper extremity splinted across her waist.

ROM, range of motion; ROS, review of systems.

relying on objective clinical examination findings for the same conditions *(12)*. CRPS most commonly begins after a sprain/strain, fracture, surgery, or period of limb immobilization *(13,14)*. Type I CRPS (previously called "reflex sympathetic dystrophy") is diagnosed with no clear nerve injury precipitating the symptoms, as in Ms. Olds. Type II CRPS (previously called "causalgia") occurs after injury to a specific large nerve. The terms *sympathetically maintained pain* and *sympathetically mediated pain* were also applied to this same symptom complex; however, sympathetic blocks are not always beneficial, especially in patients with more long-standing symptoms. As seen in

Table 6
Targeted Treatment of De Quervain's Tenosynovitis

	Nonmedication	Medication
• Restorative treatment	○ Surgical decompression	○ Local steroid injections
• Preventive therapies	○ Splints ○ Avoid repetitive wrist twisting, grasping, or pinching	○ None
• Flare techniques	○ Ice	○ Anti-inflammatory analgesics

Ms. Olds, long-lasting CPRS symptoms may extend beyond the area of original injury.

2. TREATING HAND PAIN

Disease-specific restorative treatments may be used to treat De Quervain's tenosynovitis and carpal tunnel syndrome that have not responded to conservative therapy. Long-term chronic pain management was used in each of these three patients.

2.1. De Quervain's Syndrome

De Quervain's syndrome typically responds to conservative therapy with nonsteroidal anti-inflammatory drugs (NSAIDs), splints, and/or local steroid injections (Table 6). A large, retrospective study evaluated treatment outcome from conservative therapy for De Quervain's syndrome based on initial symptom severity ($N = 300$) *(15)*. NSAIDs plus splints provided complete relief for 88% with initially mild symptoms, 35% with moderate symptoms, and 25% with severe symptoms. Injections relieved symptoms in 100% with mild symptoms, 80% with moderate symptoms, and 76% with severe symptoms. Surgical decompression is rarely needed and is typically reserved for patients failing to achieve adequate relief from more conservative measures.

De Quervain's syndrome occurring during pregnancy or lactating is typically self-limited and should be treated conservatively. One study randomized pregnant and nursing mothers with De Quervain's syndrome to either a local steroid injection into the tendon sheath or thumb spica splints *(3)*. All nine patients receiving injections reported symptom resolution 1 to 6 days after injection. In one of these women originally treated during her fifth month of pregnancy, symptoms returned when she began nursing and again resolved with a second steroid injection. Nine patients treated with splinting reported good pain relief while wearing the splint, but return of symptoms

---

Box 1
Educational Flyer for De Quervain's Syndrome

What is De Quervain's syndrome?

In 1895, a Swiss doctor named Fritz de Quervain wrote a paper describing a pain syndrome involving the tendons in the wrist. Tendons are fiber bands that connect muscles to bones. When the muscles contract, these fibers pull on the bones. This causes your joints to move. The muscles that move your hand muscles are in your forearm. The tendons for these muscles travel through the wrist in compartments or tunnels. One tunnel contains tendons for two muscles that move the thumb. Injury to the wrist or repetitive wrist motions (such as unscrewing jar lids or using a screwdriver or hammer) can cause swelling or inflammation in this tunnel. Diabetes, thyroid disease, rheumatoid arthritis, and pregnancy may also cause inflammation in this tunnel. The swelling irritates the tendons and causes pain. De Quervain's syndrome causes a pain at the base of your thumb, which may travel into the wrist and forearm. This pain will be worse when you move your thumb or wrist.

How is De Quervain's syndrome treated?

De Quervain's syndrome is treated like other types of acute inflammation:

• Rest the thumb and wrist by avoiding activities that cause pain. Sometimes a splint is used to help rest the thumb and wrist.
• Take drugs that reduce inflammation, such as Motrin® (ibuprofen) or Naprosyn® (naproxen).
• Cortisone is a powerful injectable anti-inflammatory drug. Your doctor may also help reduce the swelling by injecting cortisone into your wrist.
• Rarely, some people need to have surgery to release the trapped tendons.

Where can I learn more about De Quervain's syndrome?

Good information about De Quervain's syndrome and its treatment can be found at these websites:

• http://www.arthritisissues.com/ms/ency/565/main.html
• http://www.vandemarkortho.com/patient/pated/ctd/dqt/dgt.html
• http://my.webmd.com/content/article/78/95632.htm

---

when the splint was removed. In eight of these women, symptoms resolved spontaneously 2 to 6 weeks after they stopped breastfeeding. The other woman reported persistent pain, which responded well to a steroid injection.

Mrs. Miller was provided with an educational flyer on De Quervain's syndrome (Box 1), prescribed Motrin® (ibuprofen), and fitted with a thumb splint. She returned to the clinic in 3 weeks reporting worsening pain and difficulty wearing the splint because it interfered with activities. She was treated with a local injection of methylprednisolone and reported good symptomatic relief 3

Table 7
Targeted Treatment of Carpal Tunnel Syndrome

	Nonmedication	Medication
• Restorative treatment	○ Surgical decompression	○ Local steroid injections
• Preventive therapies	○ Nighttime wrist splints	○ None
	○ Avoid repetitive wrist flexion or extension	
• Flare techniques	○ Postural correction	○ Anti-inflammatory analgesics

days later. She continued to avoid overusing her thumb, using aides to remove jar lids and asking her older child to pick up her own toys. She successfully nursed her baby for the next several months without a return of her symptoms.

2.2. Carpal Tunnel Syndrome

Postural correction and nighttime splints typically improve carpal tunnel symptoms (Table 7). Local steroid injections may also be considered, especially when motor loss is present. Patients who are not candidates for injections may benefit from iontophoresis with corticosteroids. Physical therapists adminstering iontophoresis use electric current to deliver topically applied medications to soft tissues. A prospective study in 30 patients randomized to either corticosteroid iontophoresis every other day for 1 week or a single steroid injection showed benefit from both treatments, although injection led to superior improvement *(16)*. Pain reduction 2 and 8 weeks after treatment, respectively, were 29 and 51% with iontophoresis and 27 and 71% with injection. The number of patients experiencing paresthesia decreased between pretreatment and 8 weeks after therapy, respectively, from 96 to 35% with iontophoresis and 95 to 15% with steroid injection.

Two recent studies compared outcome in patients experiencing carpal tunnel syndrome for less than 1 year who were prospectively randomized to treatment with one to two steroid injections or surgical decompression. In one study (N = 50), improvement in symptoms and nerve conduction occurred in patients with either treatment, although benefits were greater with surgery than after a single steroid injection *(17)*. In this same study, grip strength improved in patients receiving injections, and worsened slightly after surgery. In a similar study (N = 101), injections produced better short-term symptomatic relief and comparable long-term results to surgical decompression *(18)*. In this second study, patients could receive a second injection after 2 weeks, with 84% receiving two injections. These studies suggest that both injections and surgical decompression effectively relieve carpal tunnel symptoms; however, injections may pro-

---

Box 2
Educational Flyer for Carpal Tunnel Syndrome

What is carpal tunnel syndrome?

The nerves and muscles in your arm go into your hand by traveling in tunnels in the wrist. The word carpal comes from the Greek word *karpos*, meaning "wrist." Therefore, the *carpal tunnel* is a major tunnel in your wrist. The carpal tunnel is the passageway for several tendons and the median nerve. The tendons are fiber bands that connect the muscles in your forearm to the muscles in your hand. When these muscles contract, the tendons pull on the bones and bend them at the joint. This gives you the strength and fine motions in your hand and fingers. The median nerve supplies the sensation over half of your palm on the side of your thumb and the muscles that move the thumb. Injury to the wrist or prolonged wrist strain (as can occur with scrubbing floors, driving, or resting your wrists on the desk while you type) can cause swelling or inflammation in this tunnel. Diabetes, thyroid disease, rheumatoid arthritis, and pregnancy may also cause fluid retention or inflammation in this tunnel. The swelling pinches and irritates the median nerve, causing pain and numbness over your thumb, index, and sometimes middle and ring fingers. Less commonly, people develop weakness in the thumb or a weak grip. Carpal tunnel pain is often aggravated at night.

How is carpal tunnel treated?

Carpal tunnel syndrome is treated like other types of acute inflammation:

• Rest the wrist by avoiding activities that cause pain, especially bending your wrist down or back. Sometimes a splint is used to help maintain a good wrist posture, especially at night.
• Take drugs that reduce inflammation, such as Motrin® (ibuprofen) or Naproxen® (naprosyn).
• Cortisone is a powerful injectable anti-inflammatory drug. Your doctor may also help reduce the swelling by injecting cortisone into your wrist.
• Rarely, some people need to have surgery to release the trapped nerve.

Where can I learn more about carpal tunnel syndrome?

Good information about carpal tunnel syndrome and its treatment can be found at these websites:

• http://familydoctor.org/023.xml
• http://www.medicinenet.com/carpal_tunnel_syndrome/article.htm

---

duce better results when patients are offered a second injection after 2 weeks rather than using only a single injection.

Carpal tunnel symptoms usually resolve after delivery. A survey of 46 women developing carpal tunnel syndrome with pregnancy reported persistent symptoms in only 18 patients (39%) 1 month postpartum and 2 (4%) 1 year postpartum *(10)*. Decompressive surgery was required in only two of these women. Mrs.

Table 8
Targeted Treatment of Complex Regional Pain Syndrome

	Nonmedication	Medication
• Restorative treatment	○ Physical therapy ○ Occupational therapy ○ Exercise	○ Oral steroid or sympathetic blocks for early CRPS ○ Topical DMSO ○ Possible spinal cord stimulation
• Preventive therapies	○ Physical therapy ○ Occupational therapy ○ Exercise ○ Cognitive restructuring ○ Relaxation	○ Antidepressants ○ Anti-epileptics
• Flare techniques	○ Relaxation	○ Analgesics

Do *not* splint the painful extremity in CRPS.
DMSO, dimethylsulfoxide; CRPS, complex regional pain syndrome.

Nealy was given an educational flyer explaining carpal tunnel syndrome (Box 2) and counseled that carpal tunnel symptoms generally resolve after delivery, precluding the need for surgical decompression. She was referred to a physical therapist for hand posture instruction at home and at work and application of nighttime wrist splints. NSAIDs were not prescribed because they are associated with premature closure of the fetal ductus arteriosus in the third trimester, with their use generally restricted after gestational week 32 *(19–21)*. Her symptoms abated after 2 weeks and did not return postpartum.

2.3. Complex Regional Pain Syndrome

CRPS tends to improve over time and with treatment *(12,14)*. Although frequently discussed in older literature, it is now uncommon for patients with CRPS to develop severe limb deformities, possibly as a result of better early syndrome recognition and increased awareness that increasing limb mobility is the hallmark of treatment. CRPS is treated with the combination of medications for symptomatic relief and physical rehabilitation to prevent progression to motor changes, such as reduced range of motion, joint contracture, and motor loss (Table 8). Treatment during the first few weeks of experiencing CRPS includes oral corticosteroids (30 mg daily for 2 weeks, followed by a tapering schedule) and sympathetic ganglion blocks or intravenous regional Bier blocks *(22)*. Topical cream with 50% dimethylsulfoxide also reduces symptoms in early CRPS *(23,24)*. These therapies are combined with vigorous physical therapy. The goal of early intervention with steroids and/or blocks is to provide temporary symptomatic reduction to allow optimization of participation in rehabilitative therapies. The primary treatment for both early and late CRPS is physical and occupational therapy to maintain or improve range of motion and maximize active use of the painful extremity. Gait training is essential to develop a normal, unrestricted walking pattern and a symmetrical arm swing. Psychological pain management can improve compliance with physical exercise and add skills to reduce pain. Anti-epileptics, antidepressants, and long-acting opioids may also be used to reduce allodynia or pain to improve patient cooperation with increased physical use of the painful extremity. Spinal cord stimulation may be considered for recalcitrant patients *(25)*.

Ms. Miller read an educational flyer describing CRPS (Box 3) and was educated by both the nurse practitioner and physical therapist about the importance of regaining normal use of the painful arm for improving her symptoms of CRPS. She was scheduled for a sympathetic block, followed immediately by physical therapy, so that treatment could commence when pain had been temporarily relieved by the block. The physical therapist instructed Ms. Miller in a home exercise program, and she was encouraged to resume a more normal arm swing with walking, a nonsplinted posture when she was sitting, and some normal use of the right hand, such as with eating and answering the telephone. She attended regular physical therapy sessions to reinforce arm use. Neurontin® (gabapentin) was added to help diminish allodynia. After several months, she had achieved more normal use of her right upper extremity and hand, with decreased pain complaints. She was also no longer reporting changes in hand temperature and color.

3. SUMMARY

Most common hand pain syndromes are caused by musculoskeletal or neuropathic dysfunction. Many syndromes can be readily identified at the bedside by observing patient behavior (such as extreme guarding with CRPS) and performing simple physical examination tests. Physical and occupational therapists provide essential instruction and rehabilitation for most patients with hand pain to minimize pain and disability.

REFERENCES

1. Urwin M, Symmons D, Allison T, et al. Estimating the burden of musculoskeletal disorders in the community: the comparative prevalence of symptoms at different anatomical sites, and the relation to social deprivation. Ann Rheum Dis 1998;57: 649–655.
2. Walker-K, Palmer KT, Reading I, Coggon D, Cooper C. Prevalence and impact of musculoskeletal disorders of the upper limb in the general population. Arthritis Care Res 2004;51:642–651.
3. Avci S, Yilmaz C, Sayli U. Comparison of nonsurgical treatment measures for de Quervain's disease of pregnancy and lactation. J Hand Surg (Am) 2002;27A:322–324.

Box 3
Educational Flyer for CRPS

What is complex regional pain syndrome?

After an injury, people sometimes develop a variety of persistent unpleasant sensations in the previously injured area. Long after healing occurs, a previously injured arm or leg may become very sensitive to light touch and have flare-ups with changes in temperature (usually cold), redness, and swelling. The pain is often burning and severe. Over time, you may also develop thickening of the skin, brittleness and deformity of the nails, and loss of extremity hair. These changes are complex and usually affect one area or region of the body (usually an arm or leg). This group of symptoms is, therefore, called *complex regional pain syndrome*, or *CRPS*. CRPS typically occurs after nerve trauma, fractures, sprains, and periods of immobilization or casting of an arm or leg.

Although many people have never heard of CRPS, this was first described by doctors treating soldiers for battle injuries during the Civil War. This condition was first called causalgia from the Greek word *kausos* (meaning "fever" or "burning") and *algo* (meaning "pain"). Later, doctors noted these patients had an overactive sympathetic nervous system, which controls automatic body functions, including the amount of blood that flows to your arms and legs. This causes blood flow to decrease in an arm or leg, leading to coldness and changes in the skin, nails, and hair. This led to the use of the terms *reflex sympathetic dystrophy* and *sympathetically mediated pain*. Not all patients have these sympathetic changes, so doctors now use the term CRPS.

How is CRPS treated?

People with CRPS do not like to move or have anything touch their painful arm or leg. The most important treatment, however, is to begin moving and using this painful limb.

• Do not splint your arm or leg.
• Move your arms and legs normally when you are sitting or walking.
• Work with a physical or occupational therapist to gradually regain your function. Make sure your therapist gives you a home program. Your symptoms will not get better if you move at the therapist's office, but then keep your painful arm or leg inactive once you get home. Many patients with CRPS prefer exercising in a swimming pool.

Sometimes the pain is so unbearable that you cannot stand to move your arm or leg. In this case, your doctor may inject an anesthetic medication around the nerves for your arm or leg to temporarily reduce the pain so you can start therapy. Nerve pain medications, such as Neurontin® (gabapentin) and the antidepressant medications (e.g., Elavil® and Tofranil®), can also help lessen the pain.

Where can I learn more about CRPS?

Good information about CRPS and its treatment can be found at these websites:

• http://familydoctor.org/238.xml
• http://www.rsds.org/

4. Eogan M, O'Brien C, Carolan D, Fynes M, O'Herlihy C. Median and ulnar nerve conduction in pregnancy. Int J Gynaecol Obstet 2004;87:233–236.
5. Bruske J, Bednarski M, Grzelec H, Zyluk A. The usefulness of Phalen test and the Hoffmann-Tinel sign in the diagnosis of carpal tunnel syndrome. Acta Orthop Belg 2002;68:141–145.
6. Priganc VW, Henry SM. The relationship among five common carpal tunnel syndrome tests and the severity of carpal tunnel syndrome. J Hand Ther 2003;16: 225–236.
7. Gell N, Werner RA, Franzblau A, Ulin SS, Armstrong TJ. A longitudinal study of industrial and clerical workers: incidence of carpal tunnel syndrome and assessment of risk factors. J Occup Rehabil 2005;15:47–55.
8. Bahrami MH, Rayegani SM, Fereidouni M, Baghbani M. Prevalence and severity of carpal tunnel syndrome (CTS) during pregnancy. Electromyogr Clin Neurophysiol 2005;45:123–125.
9. Padua L, Aprile I, Caliandro P, et al. Symptoms and neurophysiological picture of carpal tunnel syndrome in pregnancy. Clin Neurophysiol 2001;112:1946–1951.
10. Turgut F, Cetinsahinahin M, Turgut M, Bolukbasi O. The management of carpal tunnel syndrome in pregnancy. J Clin Neurosci 2001;8:332–334.
11. Merskey H, Bogduk N. Classification of Chronic Pain. Seattle,WA: IASP Press, 1994.
12. Galer BS, Bruehl S, Harden RN. Diagnostic clinical criteria for CRPS and painful diabetic neuropathy. Clin J Pain 1998;14:48–54.
13. Allen G, Galer BS, Schwartz L. Epidemiology of complex regional pain syndrome: a retrospective chart review of 134 patients. Pain 1999;80:539–544.
14. Sandroni P, Benrud-Larson LM, McClelland RL, Low PA. Complex regional pain syndrome type I: incidence and prevalence in Olmstead county, a population-based study. Pain 2003;103:199–207.
15. Lane LB, Boretz RS, Stuchin SA. Treatment of de Quervain's disease: role of conservative management. J Hand Surg (Br) 2001;26B:3:258–260.
16. Gökofülu F, Findikofülu G, Yorgancofülu ZR, et al. Evaluation of iontophoresis and local corticosteroid injection in the treatment of carpal tunnel syndrome. Am J Phys Med Rehabil 2005;84:92–96.
17. Hui AF, Song S, Leung CH, et al. A randomized controlled trial of surgery vs steroid injection for carpal tunnel syndrome. Neurology 2005;64:2074–2078.
18. Ly-Pen D, Andréu J, de Blas G, Sánchez-Olaso A, Millán I. Surgical decompression versus local steroid injection in carpal tunnel syndrome. A one-year, prospective, randomized, open, controlled clinical trial. Arthritis Rheum 2005;52: 612–619.
19. Momma K, Hagiwara H, Konishi T. Constriction of fetal ductus arteriosus by non-steroidal anti-inflammatory drugs: study of additional 34 drugs. Prostaglandins 1984;28:527–536.
20. Rein AJ, Nadjari M, Elchalal U, Nir A. Contraction of the fetal ductus arteriosus induced by diclofenac. Case report. Fetal Diagn Ther 1999;14:24–25.
21. Zenker M, Klinge J, Kruger C, Singer H, Scharf J. Severe pulmonary hypertension in a neonate caused by premature closure of the ductus arteriosus following maternal treatment with diclofenac: a case report. J Perinat Med 1998;26:231–234.

22. Chung OY, Bruehl SP. Complex regional pain syndrome. Curr Treatment Options Neurol 2003;5:499–511.
23. Zuurmond WA, Langendijk PJ, Bezemer PD, et al. Treatment of acute reflex sympathetic dystrophy with DMSO 50% in a fatty cream. Acta Anaesthesiol Scand 1996;40:364–367.
24. Perez RM, Zuurmond WA, Bezemer PD, et al. The treatment of complex regional pain syndrome type I with free radical scavengers: a randomized controlled study. Pain 2003;102:297–307.
25. Grabow TS, Tella PK, Raja SN. Spinal cord stimulation for complex regional pain syndrome: an evidence-based medicine review of the literature. Clin J Pain 2003;19:371–383.

8
Pain in the Foot

CHAPTER HIGHLIGHTS

- Disabling foot pain affects about 10% of adults.
- Common causes of foot pain can be distinguished by pain location, response to walking, and physical examination findings.
- Plantar fasciitis is the most common cause of heel pain.
- Painful peripheral neuropathy affects about one-fifth of all patients with diabetes.

* * *

This morning, you have four new patients with diabetes with chief complaints of a *pain in the foot*. They are all here for an initial evaluation. Here are the stories each patient tells your nurse:

Patient 1: Ms. Harvey is a 55-year-old waitress. "I just live on my feet. I've always been a morning person, but now I dread getting up. The minute my foot hits the floor, I'm in agony!"

Patient 2: Mrs. Inwood is a 65-year-old art teacher. "I know this sounds crazy, but my feet feel like they're freezing and on fire at the same time. They even bother me when I'm just lying in bed at night. They're so cold all the time; I wear thick socks even in the warm weather. When I get looks, I just tell people I'm an eccentric artist."

Patient 3: Ms. Johnson is a 19-year-old college student. "I think I've become my grandmother! I've always been an athlete, running at least 5 miles each morning and evening. I really pushed myself this spring so I'd be in great shape this summer, and now I can't even walk!"

Patient 4: Mrs. Klein is a 48-year-old secretary. "Every time I walk it hurts. The other day when I went to buy new shoes, the sale clerk suggested I switch to a "sensible" shoe. You should have seen the old lady shoes she tried to sell me!"

From: *Current Clinical Practice: Headache and Chronic Pain Syndromes: The Case-Based Guide to Targeted Assessment and Treatment*
By: D. A. Marcus © Humana Press, Totowa, NJ

Table 1
Common Causes of Chronic Foot Pain

Disease category	Specific diseases
• Musculoskeletal	○ Plantar fasciitis
	○ Arthritis and joint disease
	(e.g., rheumatoid arthritis, bunions, gout)
• Neuropathic	○ Peripheral neuropathy
	○ Compressive neuropathy (e.g., tarsal tunnel syndrome)
	○ Neuroma
• Vascular	○ Peripheral vascular disease
• Dermatological	○ Corns
	○ Calluses
	○ Nail disorders

1. EVALUATING FOOT PAIN

A survey of almost 5000 adults seeing general practitioners noted foot pain lasting at least 1 day during the preceding month in 20% of men and 24% of women *(1)*. Current disabling foot pain was identified in 8% of men and 11% of women. Only 36% of those reporting disabling foot pain had received medical attention. The prevalence of foot pain increased with age, peaking between ages 55 and 64, when disabling foot pain affects 12% of men and 15% of women. Foot pain can significantly impair walking, as well as work, sports, and other leisure activities.

Although the chief complaints and brief histories in these four patients are typical, none has provided enough information to formulate an educated diagnosis. While each patient has the same primary complaint, differences in history and examination can provide ready clues to diagnostic possibilities (Table 1). Extracting important features to distinguish among common disorders depends on a targeted evaluation that focuses on high-yield questions and examination findings to help distinguish among the many possible causes of foot pain.

1.1. Developing a High-Yield Targeted Evaluation of Foot Pain

Evaluations of patients with foot pain should be targeted to specific likely clinical scenarios to help confirm or refute clinical diagnoses (Table 2). The same evaluation principles apply to each patient regarding features in the history, physical examination findings, and the need to proceed with testing. Details of the targeted examination are outlined in Table 3. The neurological examination in patients with foot pain should include vibratory testing to effectively identify peripheral neuropathy. Ideally, the slightest vibration perceived in the great toe of the examiner should also be detected in the healthy patient's great toe. When

Table 2
Distinguishing Common Causes of Foot Pain

	Location	Unilateral versus bilateral	Response to walking
• Morton's neuroma	○ Ball of foot	○ Unilateral	○ Worse
• Peripheral neuropathy	○ Distal foot or stocking	○ Bilateral	○ Usually better
• Peripheral vascular disease	○ Diffuse foot	○ Bilateral	○ Worse
• Plantar fasciitis	○ Heel	○ Usually unilateral	○ Worse with first step; better with prolonged walking
• Tarsal tunnel syndrome	○ Medial sole and ankle	○ Unilateral	○ Worse

Table 3
Keys to a Targeted Evaluation of Foot Pain

• History	○ Clarify pain location—complete pain drawing.
	○ Identify pain descriptors—burning and numbness suggest neuropathic conditions.
	○ Note pain precipitants.
	○ Record pain provokers and pain response to walking.
	○ Identify additional medical conditions, such as diabetes, rheumatological disorders, and malignancies that suggest systemic cause of pain.
	○ Obtain complete review of systems.
• Physical examination	○ Vascular evaluation
	▪ Include temperature and color
	○ Musculoskeletal exam
	▪ Identification of joint deformities or cutaneous abnormalities (e.g., corns, warts, calluses), ROM, palpation of bones and tendinous insertions.
	○ Neurological exam
	▪ Gait examination and strength and sensory testing, including vibration.
• Testing	○ Imaging studies, including X-ray and MRI when history suggests trauma, fracture, infection, or mass lesions.
	○ NCS/EMG for peripheral or compressive neuropathy.
	○ Doppler ankle/brachial pressure index for vasculopathy.

MRI, magnetic resonance imaging; NCS/EMG, nerve conduction studies/electromyography; ROM, range of motion.

testing elderly patients or patients with diabetes, peripheral neuropathy may be suspected when vibration that is perceived in the examiner's great toe is no longer perceived at the patient's lateral malleolus.

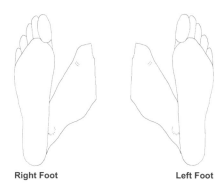

Right Foot   Left Foot

Fig. 1. Pain drawing for patients with foot pain. Patients are instructed to place an "X" at the area of maximum pain. Also, they should shade all painful areas using the following key: //// = pain; :::::: = numbness; **** = burning or hypersensitivity.

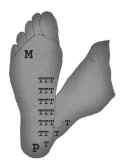

Fig. 2. Location of common unilateral foot pain syndromes. M, Morton's neuroma; P, plantar fasciitis; T, tarsal tunnel syndrome. (Reprinted with permission from ref. *1a.*)

1.2. Applying the Targeted Exam to Each Patient

Pain drawings for each patient revealed only pain in the foot or feet. In patients with pain in the feet only, a supplemental pain drawing (Fig. 1) may be used to better clarify the location and quality of the foot pain. Pain location is characteristic for several common chronic foot pain conditions (Fig. 2). The results of the targeted evaluation for each patient are provided in Tables 4 to 7. Read each patient's findings, decide if additional testing is necessary, and formulate a likely diagnosis. Then read the following sections to compare your interpretations with the patients' diagnoses in the clinic.

Table 4
Results of Targeted Evaluation for Patient No.1:
Ms. Harvey—55-Year-Old Waitress

Targeted assessment	Findings
History	○ Pain is in her left heel.
	○ Pain is severe and sharp, "like a knife cutting through my foot. I'm sure my heel bone's broken."
	○ Pain began without any trauma and is slowly getting more severe.
	○ Pain is most severe when she first gets out of bed, then lessens by the time she has dressed and walks downstairs for breakfast. It comes back every time she is off her feet for a break during the day.
	○ ROS: type 2 diabetes managed with oral hypoglycemic, obesity, mild hypercholesterolemia, and mild foot drop after hysterectomy 1 year ago.
Physical exam	
• Vascular	○ Good color and temperature; normal pulses
• Musculoskeletal	○ No obvious joint deformities or cutaneous abnormalities. Left foot dorsiflexion reproduces pain. Dorsiflexion of right foot is restricted with no pain report. Severe tenderness when palpating left medial calcaneal tubercle.
• Neurological	○ Normal neurological examination, except for minimally decreased left foot dorsiflexion.

ROM, range of motion; ROS, review of systems.

1.2.1. Patient 1: Ms. Harvey—55-Year-Old Waitress (Table 4)

Ms. Harvey's pain involves her left heel, with severe tenderness to palpation over the anterior aspect of her calcaneus. Her pain is also reproduced by dorsiflexing the foot (Fig. 3); other movements of the ankle and foot do not cause pain. Foot inspection, vascular, and neurological examinations are unremarkable, except for a mild, chronic foot drop. No additional testing is ordered.

Ms. Harvey's report of severe, nontraumatic heel pain, with maximal pain experienced on the first steps in the morning is typical of plantar fasciitis, a common cause of foot pain and the most common cause of severe heel pain. Patients with plantar fasciitis typically report their pain is at its worst when they first try to get out of bed in the morning and is aggravated after prolonged sitting. The National Ambulatory Medical Care Survey and National Hospital Ambulatory Medical Care Survey for 1995 to 2000 identified more than 1 million patient visits annually in the United States for plantar fasciitis *(2)*. Plantar fasciitis is experienced as an excruciating heel pain that increases when the foot is kept in a plantar flexed position, as occurs during sleep. When the foot is first dorsiflexed, such as when getting up out of bed in the morning, the pain is unbearable. Once the area has been stretched, as occurs with repeated foot dorsiflexion or with prolonged walking, the pain lessens.

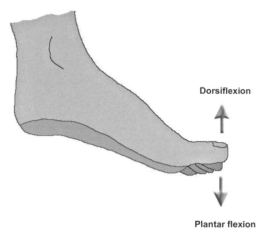

Dorsiflexion

Plantar flexion

Fig. 3. Foot flexion. Dorsiflexion occurs with bending the foot up or heel walking. Plantar flexion occurs with bending the foot down or walking on the toes.

Every time the foot rests, such as with sitting or going to bed, the area tightens, and severe pain is experienced again with the first step. A matched, case-controlled study identified obesity, spending most of the workday on one's feet, and reduced ankle dorsiflexion of both the affected and even the unaffected foot as independent risk factors for plantar fasciitis *(3)*. Plantar fasciitis is common in runners, dancers, and individuals with foot pronation. Ms. Harvey experienced a compressive peroneal neuropathy during her hysterectomy 1 year ago, with a resultant mild foot drop. Foot drop results in both reduced foot dorsiflexion and excessive pronation, both of which increase the risk for developing plantar fasciitis.

As with Ms. Harvey, radiographic studies in patients with plantar fasciitis symptoms are generally reserved for patients who fail to respond to conservative therapy. About half of those with plantar fasciitis will have heel spurs on X-ray, although these are generally unrelated to their pain symptoms. Magnetic resonance imaging (MRI) scans in plantar fasciitis typically show edema and thickening of the plantar fascia. In severe cases, tears may also be detected with MRI.

1.2.2. Patient 2: Mrs. Inwood—65-Year-Old Art Teacher (Table 5)

Mrs. Inwood describes bilateral, diffuse foot pain associated with allodynia (the perception of increased pain with sensations). Although she reports "coldness" in her feet, her pulse, coloration, and skin temperature suggest good vascularization. No musculoskeletal abnormalities are identified. No additional testing is ordered.

Table 5
Results of Targeted Evaluation for Patient 2:
Mrs. Inwood—65-Year-Old Teacher

Targeted assessment	Findings
History	○ Pain affects both feet diffusely below the ankles. ○ Pain is burning and tingling. ○ Pain has slowly developed over the last year. No preceding trauma. ○ Worst pain occurs at night when lying in bed. ○ Pain usually is less noticeable when she is walking, although it comes right back once she stops walking. ○ ROS: type 2 diabetes, well controlled until 1 year ago when she divorced and switched jobs. "I've been under too much stress and depressed to watch my diet and medicine. Things should get back to normal soon." Treated with tricyclic antidepressants after her divorce, which caused excessive sedation. Otherwise, controlled hypertension.
Physical exam • Vascular • Musculoskeletal	 ○ Good color and temperature; normal pulses ○ No obvious joint deformities or cutaneous abnormalities. Full ROM of foot and ankle. Firm palpation not more bothersome than light touch.
• Neurological	○ Normal gait and strength testing. Absent ankle reflexes bilaterally. No numbness, but reports light touch and pin prick are very bothersome diffusely in both feet. Vibration felt at examiner's toe is not perceived at the patient's great toe or ankle. Vibration is only felt when the tuning fork is so strong that an audible sound can be heard.

ROM, range of motion; ROS, review of systems.

Mrs. Inwood is diagnosed with peripheral neuropathy, which is typically described as a burning pain that is aggravated by sensory stimulation, such as light touch, cold, or vibration. Like many patients with peripheral neuropathy, Mrs. Inwood does not describe her feet as numb or lacking sensation, but reports allodynia. In patients with peripheral neuropathy, allodynia frequently results in complaints of intense foot pain with changes in temperature or light touch, such as bedclothes brushing against the feet. Patients will also often report an unnatural cold perception to the foot or a feeling that the feet are "dead." Walking may either improve or aggravate neuropathic pain, although pain is usually better with walking and worse when lying in bed. Unlike a mononeuropathy or compressive neuropathy, which is usually unilateral, most cases of peripheral neuropathy produce bilateral symptoms. Early symptoms occur distally. As neuropathy progresses, patients will develop the characteristic "stocking"-area pain and sensory loss.

Peripheral neuropathy occurs in a variety of medical illnesses, including endocrine, rheumatological, liver, kidney, infectious, malignant, and nutritional disorders. A survey of patients seeing primary care doctors identified chronic painful peripheral neuropathy in the lower extremity in 5% of nondiabetics and 17% of patients with diabetcs *(4)*. Interestingly, patients with diabetes with and without peripheral neuropathy shared similar diabetes type and duration of illness, glycemic control, and vascular risk factors. Also of note, 39% of the patients with diabetes with neuropathy had never received treatment for neuropathic pain, including 12% who had not consulted for their pain. A large, prospective, longitudinal survey evaluated more than 3000 patients with type 1 diabetes (average age = 33 years) with an initial assessment and follow-up after 6 to 10 years *(5)*. At baseline, 29% of patients had neuropathy. Of those without neuropathy at the initial assessment, neuropathy developed by the time of the follow-up (average time = 7 years) in 24%. In these patients, longer duration of type 1 diabetes, poor blood sugar control, cardiovascular risk factors, and smoking were all independent predictors for developing neuropathy at follow-up. Obesity has also been linked to increased risk for neuropathy in patients with type 1 diabetes *(6)*. Another large survey identified peripheral neuropathy in 60% of 866 patients with type 2 diabetes (average age = 57 years) attending a diabetic clinic. This survey similarly linked longer duration of type 2 diabetes and poor blood sugar control to increased risk for neuropathy *(7)*.

The diagnosis of peripheral neuropathy may be confirmed using nerve conduction studies. Nerve testing is typically reserved for patients when there is no apparent cause for peripheral neuropathy, the diagnosis cannot be clearly confirmed on clinical examination, or compressive neuropathies or other neurological conditions are considered in the differential diagnosis.

1.2.3. Patient 3: Ms. Johnson—19-Year-Old Student (Table 6)

Ms. Johnson's foot pain began after overuse, with an aggressive workout schedule before her long summer backpacking trip. She describes a neuropathic pain over her ankle and arch, with no mechanical or vascular abnormalities. No additional testing was ordered.

Ms. Johnson's history and examination are characteristic of a compressive neuropathy of the posterior tibial nerve known as tarsal tunnel syndrome. As seen in Ms. Johnson, this pain may be reproduced by percussing the posterior tibial nerve behind the medial malleolus or by dorsiflexing and everting the foot. In tarsal tunnel syndrome, nerve entrapment occurs in the tunnel formed behind the medial malleolus by the flexor retinaculum (a fibrous band located between the medial malleolus and the calcaneus) (Fig. 4). Tarsal tunnel syndrome causes a vague pain and numbness over the medial ankle, heel, sole, and foot arch. This pain is caused by compression of the tibial nerve as it passes

Table 6
Results of Targeted Evaluation for Patient 3:
Ms. Johnson—19-Year-Old Student

Targeted assessment	Findings
History	○ Pain affects her right ankle, heel, and arch. Her drawing shows symbols for pain, numbness, and burning over this entire area.
	○ Pain began during the last 3 days of a 2-month-long summer backpacking trip along the Appalachian trail. There was no specific injury that occurred on this trip.
	○ "Bumping the bone inside my right ankle puts me through the roof!" Walking also aggravates her pain, which gets worse the longer she walks.
	○ ROS: type 1 diabetes, well controlled.
Physical exam	
• Vascular	○ Good color, temperature, and pulses in both feet
• Musculoskeletal	○ No obvious joint deformities or cutaneous abnormalities.
	○ Full ROM of foot and ankle. Pain was reproduced when the examiner pushed the toes and foot up and laterally. Area of point tenderness behind tibial artery. Percussion here reproduces pain.
• Neurological	○ Normal neurological examination.

ROM, range of motion; ROS, review of systems.

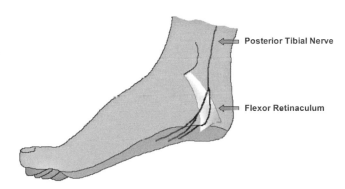

Fig. 4. Anatomy of the posterior tibial nerve. The posterior tibial nerve travels into the foot under the flexor retinaculum.

behind the medial malleolus posterior to the tibial artery. Unlike plantar fasciitis, which improves with prolonged walking, tarsal tunnel pain is aggravated by walking. In addition, percussing the flexor retinaculum may result in an electric shock-like pain, similar to percussion at the wrist for carpal tunnel syndrome.

Table 7
Results of Targeted Evaluation for Patient 4:
Mrs. Klein—48-Year-Old

Targeted assessment	Findings
History	○ Pain is located in the ball of the left foot. "It feels like I'm walking on a marble."
	○ Pain began without trauma.
	○ "Every step gives me a jolt of pain. The more I walk, the worse I feel."
	○ ROS: type 2 diabetes, controlled with diet and exercise.
Physical exam	
• Vascular	○ Good color, temperature, and pulses in both feet.
• Musculoskeletal	○ No obvious joint deformities or cutaneous abnormalities.
	○ Full ROM of foot and ankle. Palpation of the ball of the foot around the third metatarsal reproduces pain.
• Neurological	○ Normal neurological examination.

ROM, range of motion; ROS, review of systems.

Tarsal tunnel syndrome may be caused by mechanical dysfunction (including trauma), mass lesions (including varicosities, cysts, osteophytes, and tumors), and metabolic disorders causing swelling (including rheumatoid arthritis, diabetes, and thyroid disease) *(8)*. Tarsal tunnel syndrome has been reported in runners (especially after excessive training), with prolonged hiking, and after wearing compressive skates and ski boots *(9–12)*. A recent survey of long-distance backpackers identified foot numbness or paresthesias in 34% of patients *(10)*. Although most cases were considered nonspecific paresthesias, tarsal tunnel syndrome was diagnosed in 6% of those with foot symptoms. Paresthesias occurred more frequently in backpackers who were female, younger, and those hiking more than 2000 miles. In 98% of backpackers, symptoms resolved before follow-up, which occurred after an average of 1 month. Both ankle stress and hiking boot compression may contribute to the development of tarsal tunnel syndrome in hikers.

1.2.4. Patient 4: Mrs. Klein—48-Year-Old Secretary (Table 7)

Mrs. Klein's pain is located discretely in the ball of her left foot, with an electrical pain produced consistently with pressure over this area, as reported in the history and noted during the physical examination. There are no neurological, mechanical, or vascular deficits. No additional testing was ordered.

Point tenderness over the ball of the foot in Mrs. Klein is consistent with the diagnosis of Morton's neuroma. Morton's neuroma typically affects the third common digital nerve, resulting in a pain in the ball of the foot that occurs with each weight-bearing step. Walking may also cause a tingling or electric shock-

Table 8
Targeted Treatment of Plantar Fasciitis

	Nonmedication	Medication
• Restorative treatment	◦ Stretching exercises with frequent foot dorsiflexion ◦ Supportive shoes with good medial arch support ◦ Orthotics to reduce foot pronation and cushion the heel	◦ NSAIDs
• Preventive therapies	◦ Stretching exercises ◦ Supportive footwear; consider 90° night splints	◦ None
• Flare techniques	◦ Ice ◦ Stretching exercises ◦ Relaxation techniques	◦ NSAIDs ◦ Analgesics

NSAIDs, nonsteroidal anti-inflammatory drugs.

like pain around the second to fourth metatarsals. Women are more commonly affected than men. This pain will be aggravated by wearing pointed-toe, high-heel shoes. The neuroma can usually be isolated by squeezing the sides of the feet together with one hand, while pressing the ball of the foot with the other thumb. This should reproduce the pain of Morton's neuroma. Larger Morton's neuromas will usually be visible on MRI scans and ultrasound, although imaging studies are generally not necessary.

2. TREATING FOOT PAIN

Disease-specific restorative treatments may be used to treat recalcitrant tarsal tunnel syndrome and Morton's neuroma. Treating plantar fasciitis in Ms. Harvey and peripheral neuropathy in Mrs. Inwood will necessitate long-term chronic pain management. The initial treatment of tarsal tunnel syndrome and Morton's neuroma is also conservative.

2.1. Plantar Fasciitis

Although early suspicion of inflammation as the cause of plantar fasciitis led to the development of its current name, plantar fasciitis is primarily a non-inflammatory condition, caused by stress and degenerative changes in the plantar fascia and degenerative reduction in the heel pad. Treatment, therefore, focuses on stretching a shortened and stiff plantar fascia, providing arch and heel support to reduce foot pronation, and provide protective cushioning of the heel (Table 8).

A prospective study randomized 236 patients with plantar fasciitis to stretching exercises alone or stretching plus orthotics *(13)*. After 8 weeks of treatment, the outcome was superior in patients treated with prefabricated orthotics

Table 9
Targeted Treatment of Peripheral Neuropathy

	Nonmedication	Medication
• Restorative treatment	○ Management of underlying medical condition	○ Management of underlying medical condition
• Preventive therapies	○ Management of underlying medical condition	○ Antidepressants ○ Anti-epileptics
• Flare techniques	○ Aerobic exercise (walking, biking, swimming) ○ Relaxation techniques	○ Analgesics

plus stretching compared with stretching alone for both pain reduction (38% versus 29%) and percentage of patients improving with treatment (88% versus 72%).

Ms. Harvey was provided with an educational flyer on plantar fasciitis (Box 1) and advised to wear supportive footwear at all times. She was also given a heel lift wedge to elevate her medial foot slightly to prevent pronation, and was advised to consider shoe inserts to also maintain proper foot posture. She was instructed to perform stretching exercises of her Achilles tendon and plantar fascia in the morning and evening. In addition, she was instructed to avoid resting with her foot plantar-flexed, as well as advised to regularly dorsiflex her foot during the day when she was sitting and for 5 minutes in the morning before getting out of bed. After 2 weeks, her morning pain was significantly reduced. She noticed that, for the next 6 months, she needed to perform her stretching regularly to prevent the return of pain.

2.2. Peripheral Neuropathy

Peripheral neuropathy related to systemic disease may be improved by treating the primary systemic illness (Table 9). A longitudinal study comparing patients with diabetes treated with aggressive glucose management versus conventional therapy showed a reduction in the development of neuropathy of 60% during 5 years in patients treated with aggressive glucose regulation *(14)*. In addition, good blood sugar control retards the progression of peripheral neuropathy *(15)*.

Both antidepressants and anti-epileptic drugs can effectively reduce the discomfort of peripheral neuropathy. Tricyclic and dual-action antidepressants are more effective than selective serotonin reuptake inhibitors *(16)*. Gabapentin (Neurontin®) and pregabalin (Lyrica®) also effectively reduce neuropathic pain and are better tolerated than other anti-epileptics *(17)*.

Box 1
Educational Flyer for Plantar Fasciitis

What is plantar fasciitis?

Planta is the Latin word for the "bottom of your foot." The *plantar fascia* (or foot fascia) is a tough band of tissue that connects your heel bone to your toes. This band gives your arch support. With prolonged standing, excess activity, or wear and tear with aging, this band can become tight and cause pain. Plantar fasciitis gives you a severe pain on the bottom of your heel that is the worst when you first get up in the morning or after sitting for a long time. The pain usually improves with continued walking.

How is plantar fasciitis treated?

Plantar fasciitis is treated with anti-inflammatory medications (such as Motrin® or Naprosyn®), supportive shoes with good arch support, foot orthotics, and stretching exercises. Helpful orthotics will cushion the heel and prevent the foot from rolling over toward the arch. Stretching exercises should be performed frequently throughout the day. Whenever you are lying down or sitting, remember to frequently push your heels down while you pull your toes and foot up. This should cause a gentle pulling sensation in the bottom of your foot. Try to keep your ankle at a 90° angle. Avoid postures where your foot bends away from the front of your leg; for example, do not wear high heels because they hold your foot in this bad position.

When you first get up in the morning and before bed, hold an ice pack to the bottom of your foot for 10 minutes. Then do these stretches:

• Sit with your knees bent and your heels on the floor. Hold the ends of a bath towel in both hands and loop the middle under your toes. Pull the towel up toward your knees, pulling your toes up while your heels stay on the floor. Hold for 10 seconds. Relax and repeat. This stretch may initially be painful, but it should feel better after several stretches.

• Stand facing a wall. Place your painful foot 2 feet away from the wall. Place your other foot about 6 inches away from the wall. Put your hands at shoulder height against the wall and tip forward so your face is near the wall. Feel a stretch behind the calf of your painful foot. Hold 10 seconds. Relax and repeat. After several repetitions, switch feet and repeat.

• Place several small objects on the floor, such as coins, buttons, or marbles. Practice picking them up with your toes.

Where can I learn more about plantar fasciitis?

Good information about plantar fasciitis and its treatment can be found at these websites:

• http://familydoctor.org/140.xml
• http://www.aafp.org/afp/20010201/477ph.html
• http://www.intelihealth.com/IH/ihtIH?t=31156&p=~br,IHW|~st,24479|~r, WSIHW000|~b,*|

Box 2
Educational Flyer for Peripheral Neuropathy

What is peripheral neuropathy?

Neuron is the medical term for "nerve." The nerves that go to your arms, legs, hands, and feet are called the *peripheral nerves*. *Pathos* is the Greek word for "suffering." Therefore, a peripheral neuropathy is suffering or discomfort of the peripheral nerves, usually affecting the feet.

Many medical illnesses, including diabetes, thyroid disease, rheumatoid arthritis, and kidney disease, can cause damage to the peripheral nerves. This damage causes the feet to become numb, tingle, burn, or pained.

How is peripheral neuropathy treated?

In many cases, treating your medical condition will make the peripheral neuropathy better. For example, if you are a patient with diabetes, getting your blood sugar under control will help your nerves work better and will lessen the pain they are causing.

There are no medicines to improve the nerve function in peripheral neuropathy. Therefore, no medicine will get rid of your numbness. There are medicines that make the numbness less unpleasant and reduce the burning, tingling, and sensitivity that often occur with peripheral neuropathy. Medications that were originally developed to treat mood disorders (such as Elavil®, Tofranil®, and Cymbalta®) and seizures (such as Neurontin®) also reduce the unpleasant sensations of peripheral neuropathy.

Aerobic exercise can also reduce the unpleasant feeling in the feet in patients with peripheral neuropathy. Walking at least 30 minutes every other day also prevents the development of peripheral vascular disease, another common cause of painful feet in patients with diabetes and other medical illnesses.

Where can I learn more about peripheral neuropathy?

Good information about peripheral neuropathy and its treatment can be found at these websites:

• http://familydoctor.org/050.xml
• http://www.ninds.nih.gov/disorders/peripheralneuropathy/detail_peripheral neuropathy.htm

---

Mrs. Inwood was asked to meet with the nurse practitioner and dietician to help get her diabetic management under better control. She also met with a psychologist for stress management and cognitive behavioral therapy to assist with diabetic management and pain control. She was given an educational flyer about peripheral neuropathy (Box 2). Although her neuropathy pain would probably be reduced with either antidepressants or an anti-epileptic, such as gabapentin (Neurontin) or pregabalin (Lyrica), an antidepressant was selected to treat her comorbid depressive symptoms. Because of previous poor toler-

Table 10
Targeted Treatment of Tarsal Tunnel Syndrome

	Nonmedication	Medication
• Restorative treatment	○ Orthotics ○ Calf muscle-stretching exercises ○ Surgical nerve release	○ NSAIDs ○ Steroid injections into flexor retinaculum
• Preventive therapies	○ Avoid excessive exercise ○ Avoid compressive boots ○ Orthotics ○ Calf muscle-stretching exercises	○ None
• Flare techniques	○ Ice ○ Restricted exercise	○ Analgesics

NSAIDs, nonsteroidal anti-inflammatory drugs.

ability of tricyclics, she was prescribed the dual-action antidepressant duloxetine (Cymbalta®), which is an FDA-approved treatment for diabetic peripheral neuropathy, with good clinical efficacy demonstrated after 2 weeks of treatment, including for nighttime pain.

2.4. Tarsal Tunnel Syndrome

Tarsal tunnel syndrome may be effectively managed in many patients with conservative treatment that involves rest, avoidance of ankle compression, ice, and anti-inflammatory drugs (Table 10). Patients failing to achieve relief with these measures may respond to steroid injections into the flexor retinaculum. In recalcitrant patients, surgical release may be needed. A survey of tarsal tunnel release on 45 affected feet reported good to excellent relief in 60% (18).

Ms. Johnson was provided with an educational flyer (Box 3) and advised to restrict weight-bearing exercise until symptoms resolved. She was also advised to use ice and ibuprofen (Motrin®). In addition, she was cautioned about overstressing the ankle with exercise and advised to use regular stretches routinely before exercise once she resumed her regular exercise program. As is typical for backpacking-induced neuropathy, Ms. Johnson's symptoms resolved with conservative treatment during the course of approximately 3 weeks (10).

2.5. Morton's Neuroma

Morton's neuroma may initially be treated conservatively by ensuring the use of nonconstrictive footwear, restricting activities the put pressure on the ball of the foot (such as running, jumping, and dancing), and using cushioned pads under the metatarsals or orthotics to reduce pressure on the neuroma, ice, and anti-inflammatory drugs (Table 11). If these treatments are inadequately effective, local steroid injections may be helpful. Some patients will require surgical resection, which produced long-term improvement in 80% of patients

---

Box 3
Educational Flyer for Tarsal Tunnel Syndrome

What is tarsal tunnel syndrome?

Tarsos is the Greek word for "ankle." A nerve runs under a tunnel on the inside of your ankle to get to the bottom of your foot. This tunnel in your ankle is called the *tarsal tunnel.* With too much exercise or pressure on the inside of your ankle (e.g., from tight skates or hiking boots), this tunnel can get pressed and pinch the nerve that runs through it. When this nerve is pinched, you will develop a burning pain and possibly numbness in your ankle, heel, and over the sole and arch of your foot.

How is tarsal tunnel syndrome treated?

If tarsal tunnel symptoms begin after a period of ankle overuse or compression, they will usually improve with anti-inflammatory drugs (such as Motrin® or Naprosyn®), rest, ice, and wearing foot orthotics. If you are an athlete, wear good-fitting, supportive foot wear and avoid excessive training. Orthotics may also be helpful. Persistent symptoms may require a surgical release of the posterior tibial nerve that runs under the tarsal tunnel.

Where can I learn more about tarsal tunnel syndrome?

Good information about tarsal tunnel syndrome and its treatment can be found at these websites:

• http://www.medterms.com/script/main/art.asp?articlekey=11564
• http://www.footphysicians.com/info2.php?id=10

Table 11
Targeted Treatment of Morton's Neuroma

	Nonmedication	Medication
• Restorative treatment	◦ Wear roomy, comfortable shoes ◦ Orthotics and metatarsal pads	◦ NSAIDs ◦ Local steroid injections
• Preventive therapies	◦ Avoid high heels and tight or pointed-toed shoes ◦ Orthotics and metatarsal pads	◦ None
• Flare techniques	◦ Ice ◦ Metatarsal pads	◦ Analgesics

NSAIDs, nonsteroidal anti-inflammatory drugs.

---

in one series *(19)*. Repeated injections with alcohol-sclerosing therapy are effective for about 90% of patients with Morton's neuroma, with long-term relief *(20,21)*. This may provide an effective option for patients who prefer to avoid surgery. In one report, Morton's neuroma was treated in 115 patients with staged therapy consisting of education, footwear modification to wider shoes, and placement of a metatarsal pad as stage 1, local steroid plus anes-

---

Box 4
Educational Flyer for Morton's Neuroma

What is Morton's neuroma?

Neuron is the medical term for "nerve." *Oma* is the Latin word for "swelling." Therefore, a *neuroma* is a swelling or thickening around a nerve. The thickening of a neuroma is caused by repetitive minor trauma to the nerve or its surrounding structures. In 1876, Dr. Morton described a painful foot condition where a thickening occurs in the nerve going to your toes. This thickening occurs in the ball of your foot. This condition was named *Morton's neuroma*. People with Morton's neuroma often complain that they feel like they are walking on a marble. Pressing or walking on this thickening can cause a severe burning pain in your foot.

How is Morton's neuroma treated?

In many cases, Morton's neuroma is thought to occur from wearing tight-fitting shoes, especially high heels with pointed toes, which squeeze the ball of your foot. The first step to treating Morton's neuroma is to rest the foot and use ice packs. Switch to comfortable, low heeled shoes that have lots of room at the front of the foot. Wearing orthotics or pads to cushion the ball of your foot may also be helpful. Anti-inflammatory medications (such as Motrin® or Naprosyn®) are also usually helpful. If these simple measures do not help, a cortisone injection may be beneficial. In some cases, surgical removal of the neuroma will be needed.

Where can I learn more about Morton's neuroma?

Good information about Morton's neuroma and its treatment can be found at these websites:

• http://www.mayoclinic.com/invoke.cfm?objectid=CB793439-A249-45C7-B4B089DBC882B8D8
• http://www.footphysicians.com/info?.php?id=20
• http://www.intelihealth.com/IH/ihtIH?t=24456&p=~br,IHW|~st,24479|~r, WSIHW000|~b,*|

---

thetic injection as stage 2, and surgical excision as stage 3 *(22)*. Patients waited 3 months in each stage before determining efficacy and the need for additional treatment. After completing stage 1 conservative treatment, 41% of patients were satisfied with their improvement. An additional 47% of patients who failed stage 1 treatment and were treated with injections were satisfied with their relief. Only 24 patients (21%) progressed to surgery, with improvement in 23 of these postoperatively (96%).

Mrs. Klein was given an educational flyer on Morton's neuroma (Box 4) and agreed to switch her pointed-toe stilettos for a flat shoe with ample toe room, which she agreed was more comfortable and still attractive. A metatarsal pad was placed in her shoe for added cushioning. She minimized wear-bearing activities and used ice after walking, along with daily naproxen (Naprosyn®).

This provided only limited improvement, and she was treated with a local cortisone injection, with good symptomatic relief.

3. SUMMARY

Every foot pain in patients with diabetes is not necessarily caused by peripheral neuropathy or vascular disease. Although none of these four patients had peripheral arteriopathy as a cause of foot pain, peripheral vascular pain or claudication also occurs commonly in patients with diabetes. Using a Doppler ankle/brachial index less than 0.9 for diagnosis, peripheral arterial disease can be identified in about 25% of patients with diabetes *(23,24)*. Patients with vascular claudication usually describe coldness of the feet at rest, with diffuse foot aching, cramping, fatigue, and pain with walking. Other risk factors for vascular claudication include smoking, hypercholesterolemia, and hypertension. The treatment of peripheral arterial disease includes risk factor modification, antiplatelet agents, cilostazol (Pletal®) in patients without heart failure, and exercise (such as walking 30 minutes every other day). Focusing on foot pain location, quality, and response to walking helps differentiate among the common causes of chronic foot pain.

REFERENCES

1. Garrow AP, Silman AJ, Macfarlane GJ. The Cheshire Foot Pain and Disability Survey: a population survey assessing prevalence and associations. Pain 2004;110: 378–384.
1a. Marcus DA. Chronic Pain: A Primary Care Guide to Practical Management. Totowa, NJ: Humana Press, 2005.
2. Riddle DL, Schappert SM. Volume of ambulatory care visits and patterns of care for patients diagnosed with plantar fasciitis: a national study of medical doctors. Foot Ankle Int 2004;25:303–310.
3. Riddle DL, Pulisic M, Pidcoe P, Johnson RE. Risk factors for plantar fasciitis: a matched case–control study. J Bone Joint Surg Am 2003;85A:872–877.
4. Daousi C, MacFarlance IA, Woodward A, et al. Chronic painful peripheral neuropathy in an urban community: a controlled comparison of people with and without diabetes. Diabet Med 2004;21:976–982.
5. Tesfaye S, Chaturvedi N, Eaton SM, et al. Vascular risk factors and diabetic neuropathy. N Engl J Med 2005;352:341–350.
6. De Block CE, De Leeuw IH, Van Gaal LF. Impact of overweight on chronic microvascular complications in type 1 diabetic patients. Diabetes Care 2005;28:1649–1655.
7. Börü ÜT, Alp R, Sargin H, et al. Prevalence of peripheral neuropathy in Type 2 diabetic patients attending a diabetes center in Turkey. Endocrin J 2004;51:563–567.
8. Mahan KT, Rock JJ, Hillstrom HJ. Tarsal tunnel syndrome. A retrospective study. J Am Pod Med Assoc 1996;86:81–91.
9. Jackson DL, Haglund BL. Tarsal tunnel syndrome in runners. Sports Med 1992; 13:146–149.

10. Boulware DR. Backpacking-induced paresthesias. Wilderness Environ Med 2003;14:161–166.
11. Watson BV, Algahtani H, Broome RJ, Brown JD. An unusual presentation of tarsal tunnel syndrome caused by an inflatable ice hockey skate. Can J Neurol Sci 2002;29:386–389.
12. Yamamoto S, Tominaga Y, Yura S, Tada H. Tarsal tunnel syndrome with double causes (ganglion, tarsal coalition) evoked by ski boots. Case report. J Sports Med Phys Fitness 1995;35:143–145.
13. Pfeffer G, Bacchetti P, Deland J, et al. Comparison of custom and prefabricated orthoses in the initial treatment of proximal plantar fasciitis. Foot Ankle Int 1999; 20:214–221.
14. The Diabetes Control and Complications Trial Research Group. The effect of intensive treatment of diabetes on the development and progression of long–term complications in insulin-dependent diabetes mellitus. N Engl J Med 1993; 329:977–986.
15. Huang CC, Chen TW, Weng MC, et al. Effect of glycemic control on electro-physiologic changes of diabetic neuropathy in type 2 diabetic patients. Kaohsiung J Med Sci 2005;21:15–21.
16. Goodnick PJ. Use of antidepressants in the treatment of comorbid diabetes mellitus and depression as well as in diabetic neuropathy. Ann Clin Psychiatry 2001;13: 31–41.
17. Wiffen P, Collins S, McQuay H, et al. Anticonvulsant drugs for acute and chronic pain. Cochrane Database Syst Rev 2005;20:CD00113.
18. Mahan KT, Rock JJ, Hillstrom HJ. Tarsal tunnel syndrome. A retrospective study. J Am Pod Med Assoc 1996;86:81–91.
19. Ruuskanen MM, Niinimaki T, Jalovaara P. Results of the surgical treatment of Morton's neuralgia in 58 operated intermetatarsal spaces followed over 6 (2–12) years. Arch Orthop Trauma Surg 1994;113:78–80.
20. Dockery GL. The treatment of intermetatarsal neuromas with 4% alcohol sclerosing injections. J Foot Ankle Surg 1999;38:403–408.
21. Fanucci E, Masala S, Fabiano S, et al. Treatment of intermetatarsal Morton's neuroma with alcohol injection under US guide: 10 month follow-up. Eur Radiol 2004;14:514–518.
22. Bennett GL, Graham CE, Mauldin DM. Morton's interdigital neuroma: a comprehensive treatment protocol. Foot Ankle Int 1995;16:760–763.
23. Bundo M, Auba J, Valles R, et al. Peripheral arteriopathy in type 2 diabetes mellitus. Aten Primaria 1998;22:5–11.
24. Lange S, Diehm C, Darius H, et al. High prevalence of peripheral arterial disease and low treatment rates in elderly primary care patients with diabetes. Exp Clin Endocrinol Diabetes 2004;112:556–573.

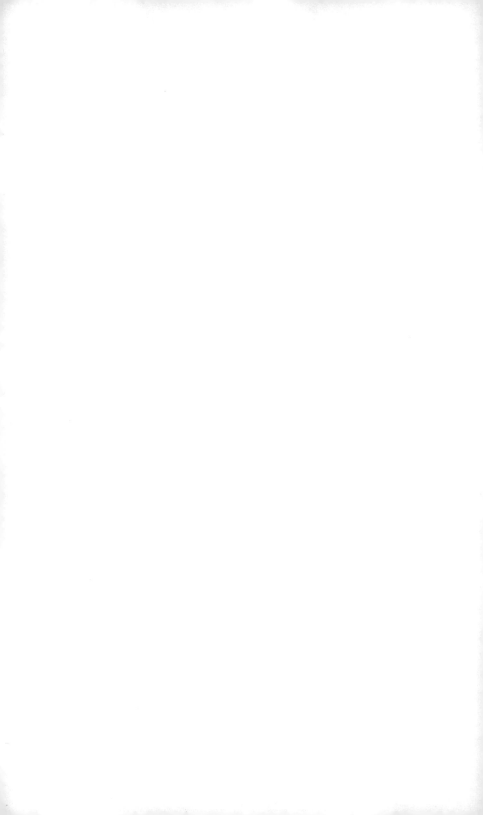

9

Pain in the Abdomen

CHAPTER HIGHLIGHTS

- Patients reporting abdominal pain should be questioned about diet, bowel habits, constitutional symptoms, and family history of gastrointestinal (GI) disease.

- In children, stomachache is usually nonspecific when the pain is located around the umbilicus and not related to changes in bowel habits, nausea, weight loss, or fever.

- Rectal and pelvic examinations should be included in the assessment of abdominal pain.

- Modifiable factors for colon cancer include obesity, inactivity, alcohol intake, cigarette smoking, and possibly dietary factors.

* * *

This morning, you have five new patients who range in age from 10 to 64 years old. Each patient comes to the office with a chief complaint of *a pain in the abdomen*. They are all here for a consultation. Here are the stories each patient tells your nurse:

Patient 1: Ms. Nichols is a 25-year-old psychologist working in an academic setting. "This belly pain is too much. I go out with my friends and head straight to the bathroom after we finish eating. My friends are all convinced I've developed bulimia. I'm starting to cut back on traveling and going out because of this embarrassing stomach pain."

Patient 2: Mr. Oliver is a 35-year old disabled construction worker. "I was disabled a couple of years ago for pain and finally got things under pretty good control. Now I've got this terrible belly pain and I can't do anything again. I stopped my exercises and walking. It's such a problem, I hate to leave the house anymore."

Patient 3: Ms. Palmer is a 42-year-old pharmaceutical representative. "It's so hard for me to keep up my job with the awful abdominal pain. I even sell gastrointestinal products, but none of them seem to work for me."

From: *Current Clinical Practice: Headache and Chronic Pain Syndromes:
The Case-Based Guide to Targeted Assessment and Treatment*
By: D. A. Marcus © Humana Press, Totowa, NJ

Patient 4: Ryan is a 10-year-old fifth grader. "I switched schools this year and it's been hard making new friends. I know my mom thinks I just make up this stomach pain so I can stay home and watch TV, but it really does hurt sometimes."

Patient 5: Mr. Schmidt is a 64-year-old retired engineer who spends several days a week out in a fishing boat with his life-long buddies. "My wife's been after me for several months to see the doctor and now the guys are sick of hearing me talk about my bowels like an old man. My wife insists everything would be cleared up if I ate less meat and more fiber, but I hate those twigs and weeds she tries to give me."

1. EVALUATING ABDOMINAL PAIN

Although the chief complaints and brief histories in these five patients are typical, none has provided enough information to formulate an educated diagnosis. Each patient has the same primary complaint; however, differences in history and examination can provide ready clues to diagnostic possibilities (Table 1). Extracting important features to distinguish among common disorders depends on a targeted evaluation that focuses on high-yield questions and examination findings that help distinguish among the many possible causes of abdominal pain.

1.1. Developing a High-Yield Targeted Evaluation of Abdominal Pain

Evaluations of patients with abdominal pain should be targeted to specific likely clinical scenarios to help confirm or refute clinical diagnoses. The same evaluation principles apply to each patient regarding features in the history, physical examination findings, and the need to proceed with testing (Table 2). In general, a history of childhood abuse, especially sexual abuse, occurs more frequently in adults with chronic pain *(1,2)*. This relationship is particularly strong in patients reporting abdominal or pelvic pain. For example, a survey of 206 consecutive patients evaluated in a university gastroenterology practice recorded prior sexual abuse in 88 patients (43%) *(3)*.

Patients with abdominal pain not clearly related to GI pathology should be screened for myofascial abdominal pain, testing for Carnett's sign. While lying supine with legs extended, the patient lifts her head and shoulders a few inches off of the examination table, causing contraction of the abdominal muscles. Aggravation of pain and tenderness of tensed muscles is a positive Carnett's sign, suggesting muscular pain. Two surveys of more than 100 patients, each with acute abdominal pain, showed the presence of Carnett's sign accurately distinguished visceral from nonvisceral pathology *(4,5)*. In addition, a pelvic examination should be included as part of the abdominal examination for all women reporting abdominal pain.

Table 1
Common Causes of Chronic or Recurring Abdominal Pain

Disease category	Specific diseases	
• Gastrointestinal	◦ Constipation ◦ Inflammatory bowel disease ◦ Lactose intolerance ◦ Tumor	◦ *Helicobacter pylori* gastritis ◦ Irritable bowel syndrome ◦ Pancreatitis
• Gynecological	◦ Endometriosis ◦ Ovarian cysts	◦ Pelvic inflammatory disease
• Musculoskeletal	◦ Myofascial abdominal wall pain	
• Neurological	◦ Abdominal migraine in kids	◦ Abdominal epilepsy in kids (rare)

Table 2
Keys to a Targeted Evaluation of Abdominal Pain

• History	◦ Clarify pain location ▪ complete pain drawing ◦ Record pain precipitants ◦ Record changes in bowel habits, relationship of pain to diet or eating, constitutional symptoms (weight change and fever), other aggravating factors ◦ Identify additional medical conditions and medication use ◦ Note family history of colon cancer or inflammatory bowel disease and history of abuse. ◦ Obtain complete review of systems, including gynecological history in women
• Physical examination	◦ Abdominal examination ▪ Auscultation, palpation, and rectal exam ◦ Gynecological examination in women ◦ Musculoskeletal exam ▪ Test for Carnett's sign ◦ Neurological exam ▪ Gait and lower extremity strength, reflexes, and sensation
• Testing	◦ Blood ▪ Blood count, chemistries, erythrocyte sedimentation rate, trypsinogen if diarrhea and steatorrhea, secretin hormone-stimulation test for suspected pancreatitis, thyroid functions, celiac sprue antibodies if diarrhea ◦ Urine ▪ Urinalysis, pregnancy test ◦ Stool ▪ Blood, plus ova and parasites if diarrhea ◦ Endoscopic retrograde cholangiopancreatography with abdominal X-ray or computed tomography for suspected pancreatitis ◦ Flexible sigmoidoscopy or colonoscopy

Table 3
Results of Targeted Evaluation for Patient 1:
Ms. Nichols—25-Year-Old Psycholgist

Targeted assessment	Findings
History	○ Pain began without injury or illness about 2 years ago. About twice a week, she gets recurrent bouts of abdominal pain, bloating, and diarrhea. Even when she has diarrhea, she still feels that she has not fully evacuated. Pain is improved after bowel movements. She also reports bloating and occasional mucus in her stool. She has about 5 to 10 days per month where she has pain and diarrhea 2 to 4 times daily. The rest of the month, she is pain free. She has not identified any particular food items, including milk products, associated with her complaints. An herbalist previously suggested a gluten-free diet, which did not improve her symptoms.
	○ No additional medical complaints or family history of gastrointestinal disease. She was molested by an uncle during elementary school, but never told an adult. She does not use any laxative or stool-binding agents. She was previously treated with two tricyclic antidepressants to improve sleep; however, they caused intolerable sedation.
	○ ROS is negative except for poor sleep and irregular menstrual periods; she is sexually active without consistent contraception.
Physical exam	
• Abdominal	○ Active bowel sounds, mild diffuse tenderness, no organomegally.
• Gynecological	○ Normal pelvic exam.
• Musculoskeletal	○ Negative Carnett's sign.
• Neurological	○ Normal gait and strength, sensation, and reflexes in the lower extremities.

ROS, review of systems.

1.2. Applying the Targeted Exam to Each Patient

Pain drawings showed pain isolated to the abdomen for all patients except for Mr. Oliver, who also describes chronic low back pain. The results of the targeted evaluation are provided for each patient in Tables 3 to 7. Assess each patient's findings, determine if additional testing is necessary, and formulate a likely diagnosis. Then read the following sections to compare your interpretations with the patients' diagnoses in the clinic.

1.2.1. Patient 1: Ms. Nichols—25-Year-Old Psycholgist (Table 3)

Ms. Nichols describes intermittent pain and diarrhea beginning without inciting event. Her symptoms are not progressive, she has no additional medical or gynecological complaints, and there is no family history of GI disease. A pregnancy test is negative. She was given a tentative diagnosis of irritable bowel syndrome (IBS), and was tested with a complete blood count, erythrocyte sedimentation rate, thyroid functions, and electrolytes, all of which were normal. Antibody testing for celiac sprue antibodies was not performed because of failure to respond to gluten restriction. History also did not support a diagnosis of lactose intolerance. Fecal testing showed no blood, ova, or parasites. A flexible sigmoidoscopy was also normal. The diagnosis of IBS was, therefore, confirmed.

IBS describes the combination of recurrent lower abdominal pain, change in bowel habits, and bloating or rectal urgency in patients without identified structural or biochemical pathology. The diagnosis of IBS has been standardized with the development of the Rome criteria, which were revised in 2000 to include requirements for 12 weeks or more of abdominal pain during the preceding year with at least two of the following symptoms: relief with bowel movement, pain onset associated with change in bowel movement frequency, and/or pain onset associated with change in stool appearance *(6)*. Additional symptoms frequently include bowel movements more than three times daily or less than three times weekly; abnormally loose or hard bowel movements; straining, urgency, or feeling of incomplete bowel evacuation; mucus in stool; bloating or abdominal distention. A large international population survey noted that symptoms of IBS occur an average of 7 days per month *(7)*. Most people reported two episodes daily, with each episode lasting about 1 hour.

1.2.2. Patient 2: Mr. Oliver—35-Year-Old Disabled Worker (Table 4)

Mr. Oliver reports abdominal pain and constipation, which began after titrating to effective dosages of two constipating medications. He has no additional medical complaints or family history of GI illness. His physical examination is remarkable for chronic left S1 radiculopathy related to his chronic low back pain. Blood work, including a complete blood count, chemistries, and thyroid functions, was normal. Stool was negative for occult blood. Mr. Oliver was tentatively diagnosed with medication-related constipation.

Constipation can become a treatment-limiting side effect with opioids, especially in patients concomitantly treated with other constipating medications, such as tricyclic antidepressants. Constipation can be reduced by adding an exercise program, fiber-rich foods, and stool softeners, as needed. A review of the literature identified reports of constipation in an average of 15% of patients with chronic nonmalignant pain treated with opioids, although the variability among trials was high *(8)*. The occurrence of constipation is also influenced by choice of opioid. In a large study of more than 1800 opioid-treated patients with pain, constipation was more likely to occur with oxycodone (6.1%) or morphine (5.1%) in comparison with transdermal fentanyl (3.7%) *(9)*. Clinical experience supports reduction in constipation when patients are switched to fentanyl.

Table 4
Results of Targeted Evaluation for Patient 2:
Mr. Oliver—35-Year-Old Disabled Worker

Targeted assessment	Findings
History	○ Pain began insidiously, without injury or illness. Progressively worse over the last 2 months.
	○ Pain is somewhat aggravated with eating any type of food, and bowel movements occur typically every 3 days. There have been no fevers or change in weight.
	○ He is also receiving treatment for chronic low back pain, with four prior surgeries, including laminectomies and one fusion. Three months ago, he began long-acting oxycodone for chronic disabling pain and amitriptyline for depression, both of which were titrated to effective dosages. He used a variety of over-the-counter laxatives, with poor success.
	○ No family history of inflammatory bowel disease. Physically and sexually abused as a child by a neighbor, who was subsequently arrested. Patient attended several sessions with a therapist after the abuse was discovered.
	○ ROS remarkable for poor sleep, mild depression, obesity, and hypertension.
Physical exam	
• Abdominal	○ Quiet belly, mild diffuse tenderness, no organomegaly.
• Musculoskeletal	○ Negative Carnett's sign.
• Neurological	○ Normal gait. Normal strength in the lower extremities, with a decreased left ankle jerk and sensation over the great toe.

ROS, review of systems.

1.2.3. Patient 3: Ms. Palmer—42-Year-Old Pharmaceutical Representative
(Table 5)

Ms. Palmer reports constant abdominal pain without a change in bowel habits or relationship to eating. Pain severity increases with maneuvers that tense the abdominal muscles. There are no additional medical or gynecological complaints or a family history of GI disease. Her examination identifies trigger points, a positive Carnett's sign, and is otherwise unremarkable. No additional testing is ordered and she is diagnosed with myofascial abdominal pain.

Myofascial abdominal wall pain should be considered in patients lacking GI or constitutional complaints, with pain aggravated by postural changes, coughing, sneezing, or deep breathing. Myofascial pain of the rectus abdominis, pyramidalis, obliques, and transversus abdominus muscles is a common cause of nonvisceral chronic abdominal pain. A total of 26% of patients referred by gastroenterologists to a pain clinic for chronic abdominal pain of unknown etiology were eventually diagnosed with myofascial abdominal pain in a retrospective chart review *(10)*.

Table 5
Results of Targeted Evaluation for Patient No. 3:
Ms. Palmer—42-Year-Old Pharmaceutical Representative

Targeted assessment	Findings
History	○ Since starting her new territory, she has abdominal pain that's present most of the time, with fluctuating severity. Pain is unchanged with eating and there are no changes in bowel habits. Pain is aggravated with getting up out of bed and coughing.
	○ General health is good. There is no fever or weight change.
	○ No family history of inflammatory bowel disease or personal history of abuse.
	○ ROS is remarkable for mild anxiety. Menstrual periods are regular; oral contraceptives are used; normal PAP smear was obtained 4 months ago.
Physical exam	
• Abdominal	○ Normal bowel sounds, mild diffuse tenderness, no organomegaly.
• Gynecological	○ Normal pelvic exam.
• Musculoskeletal	○ Diffuse areas along the lateral borders of the rectus abdominis are tender and increase pain when palpated.
	○ Positive Carnett's sign.
• Neurological	○ Normal gait and strength, sensation, and reflexes in the lower extremities.

ROS, review of systems.

1.2.4. Patient 4: Ryan —10-Year-Old Fifth Grader (Table 6)

Ryan describes nonprogressive, intermittent abdominal pain unrelated to eating. There are no bowel habit changes, no additional medical complaints, and normal growth and development. Ryan has a family history of IBS in his mother, but no inflammatory bowel disease. His physical examination is normal. No additional testing is ordered, and he is diagnosed with functional abdominal pain.

Stomach pain is very common in children. A survey of school children ages 6 to 13 years old found a prevalence of stomachache monthly in 39%, weekly in 19%, and more than once a week in 8% *(11)*. Although stomachache overall occurred more frequently in girls, reports of frequent stomachache were similar for boys and girls. Benign recurrent abdominal pain is more prevalent in children with anxiety, those who live in a single parent home, or those with a parent with GI complaints *(12)*. In addition, children with recurrent abdominal pain often also endorse other pain complaints, especially headache *(12)*. Ryan's pain is located diffusely around his umbilicus. Surveys of children with recurrent abdominal pain reveal specific abdominal pathology in 38 to 45% *(12a,13)*. A specific pathology is more likely to be present when pain is

Table 6
Results of Targeted Evaluation for Patient 4:
Ryan—10-Year-Old Student

Targeted assessment	Findings
History	○ Pain occurs around the umbilicus about twice weekly, not related to food or bowel habits. Each pain episode usually lasts less than 1 hour. ○ His general health and growth are good. ○ Ryan's mother has irritable bowel syndrome and dyspepsia. No history of abuse. ○ ROS is unremarkable expect for medical conditions. Ryan moved to a new school this year, after his parents' divorce and he seems to be adjusting well to the new situation.
Physical exam • Abdominal • Musculoskeletal • Neurological	○ Development appropriate for age. ○ Active bowel sounds, mild diffuse tenderness, no organomegaly. ○ Negative Carnett's sign. ○ Normal neurological examination.

ROS, review of systems.

located distant from the umbilicus, related to diet or eating, or associated with diarrhea, constipation, vomiting, weight loss, or fever *(14)*. Changes in growth patterns or other physical abnormalities or a family history of inflammatory bowel disease also suggest specific pathology. Most children reporting chronic abdominal pain will not need additional diagnostic testing *(15)*.

Diagnostic terminology for benign, recurring abdominal pain is in transition. In 2005, the American Academy of Pediatrics and the North American Society for Pediatric Gastroenterology, Hepatology, and Nutrition introduced the term functional abdominal pain to replace the older terminology of recurrent abdominal pain *(16)*. Functional abdominal pain includes functional dyspepsia, IBS, abdominal migraine, and functional abdominal pain syndrome (functional abdominal pain without dyspepsia, irritable bowel, or abdominal migraine.) In one survey, nearly 2 out of 3 of 107 pediatric patients with three or more episodes of recurrent abdominal pain during the preceding 3 months who did not have identified organic pathology could be assigned a functional diagnosis: IBS in 45%, functional dyspepsia 16%, functional abdominal pain 8%, and abdominal migraine 5% *(17)*.

1.2.5. Patient 5: Mr. Schmidt—64-Year-Old Retired Engineer (Table 7)

Mr. Schmidt reports a recent change in bowel habits, along with weight changes and a questionable family history. Blood work is remarkable for mild

Table 7
Results of Targeted Evaluation for Patient 5:
Mr. Schmidt—64-Year-Old Retired Engineer

Targeted assessment	Findings
History	○ Lower abdominal cramping and a sensation of needing to have a bowel movement even after evacuation is complete.
	○ 15-pound unintentional weight loss over the last 2 months. Constipation with occasional dark stools.
	○ No additional medical complaints. Over-the-counter medications have been ineffective.
	○ Brother with rectal polyp; diagnosis unknown to patient. Sister with gastric ulcers and a hiatal hernia. No history of abuse.
	○ ROS remarkable for long-standing obesity and inactivity. Wife complains that he drinks too much, but this has never interfered with work or household activities.
Physical exam	
• Abdominal	○ Active bowel sounds, no organomegaly, discomfort on rectal examination.
• Musculoskeletal	○ Negative Carnett's sign.
• Neurological	○ Normal neurological examination.

ROS, review of systems.

anemia and stool guaiac is heme-positive. A colonoscopy is performed, identifying colon cancer.

Several modifiable risk factors have been linked to increased risk for developing colon cancer, including obesity, physical inactivity, alcohol consumption, and cigarette smoking *(18,19)*. Diets low in fiber and folic acid and high in red meat may also increase colon cancer risk. Although high fiber diets seem to decrease colon cancer risk, individuals with low fiber intake typically have additional risk factors, such as low folate, low physical activity, etc., which may be stronger risk factors *(20,21)*. Data also suggest that supplemental folate and calcium may minimize colon cancer risk *(22,23)*.

2. TREATING ABDOMINAL PAIN

Disease-specific restorative treatments may be used to treat Mr. Oliver and Mr. Schmidt. Mr. Oliver was switched to fentanyl and a selective serotonin reuptake, and prescribed daily Senekot® (senna), regular morning exercise, and a high-fiber breakfast, with resultant resolution of constipation and good control of his chronic low back pain complaints. Mr. Schmidt was referred to an oncologist and treated with tumor resection and radiation. He continued to do well and was disease-free 5 years after initial treatment.

Table 8
Targeted Treatment of Irritable Bowel Syndrome

	Nonmedication	Medication
• Restorative treatment	○ None	○ None
• Preventive therapies	○ Chinese medicine ○ Relaxation ○ Cognitive–behavioral therapy	○ Tegaserod, alosetron ○ Tricyclic antidepressants ○ Peppermint oil ○ STW 5
• Flare techniques	○ Relaxation ○ Cognitive–behavioral therapy	○ Osmotic laxatives ○ Loperamide

Treating IBS in Ms. Nichols, functional abdominal pain in Ryan, and myofascial abdominal pain in Ms. Palmer will necessitate long-term chronic pain management. A review of treatment recommendations for myofascial pain is described in Chapter 5. Ms. Palmer was treated with physical therapy for abdominal muscle stretching and strengthening. She also met with an occupational therapist for training in body mechanics for transporting cases of supplies. One month after beginning to exercise and use a pull-cart for moving supplies from the car to the offices, her abdominal pain was markedly improved.

2.1. Chronic IBS

Selected treatments for IBS vary based on predominant symptoms of constipation or diarrhea (Table 8). A recent literature review of studies testing treatment efficacy in IBS identified tegaserod (Zelnorm®) and osmotic laxatives (e.g., milk of magnesia) as effective treatment for IBS with constipation *(24)*. Tricyclics, loperamide (Imodium®), and alosetron (Lotronex®) benefit patients with IBS who have diarrhea. Bulking agents were not found to be effective. Effective alternative therapy includes traditional Chinese medicine, relaxation training, cognitive–behavioral therapy, and peppermint oil *(24a,b)*. A recent double-blind, placebo-controlled study compared the efficacy of herbal therapy and placebo in 208 patients with IBS *(25)*. Patients were treated three times daily for 4 weeks with STW 5® (containing bitter candytuft, chamomile flower, peppermint leaves, caraway fruit, licorice root, lemon balm leaves, celandine herbs, angelica root, and milk thistle fruit), bitter candytuft monotherapy, or placebo. Reduction in abdominal pain score was modest and similar with bitter candytuft and placebo after 2 weeks (28%) and 4 weeks (35%). Pain reduction was significantly higher with STW 5 at both 2 (42%; $p = 0.003$) and 4 (65%; $p = 0.0009$) weeks. This study also highlights modest pain relief even with placebo, supporting the need for placebo-controlled studies to determine treat-

---

Box 1
Educational Flyer for Irritable Bowel Syndrome

What is irritable bowel syndrome?

Irritable bowel syndrome (IBS) is a common condition with bouts of abdominal pain and a change in bowel habits, such as diarrhea, constipation, or frequent bowel movements. You may have symptoms several days each month or several days each week. You may also have a couple or many bouts on the days when you are affected. Pain and need to have a bowel movement often occur right after eating. Pain usually improves after having a bowel movement, although you may feel like you still need to go to the bathroom even when you do not.

No one is sure what causes IBS. IBS does not lead to other bowel problems or colon cancer. The good news is that IBS can be managed with a combination of medication and nonmedication treatments.

How is IBS treated?

Eat a healthy diet and avoid specific foods that seem to trigger your bouts of pain. Adding soluble fiber to your diet can help improve both diarrhea and constipation. Soluble fiber can be found in oat bran and psyllium (Fiberall® or Metamucil®).

IBS often is aggravated by stress. When you experience a stressful situation, your body will react by releasing a variety of chemicals that can affect your digestive system. You will probably be more sensitive to these changes because you have IBS. Stress management can teach you ways to have your body react differently to stress so that you are less likely to release pain-provoking chemicals.

A variety of medications can also help reduce symptoms of IBS, including tricyclic antidepressants (including Elavil® and Tofranil®) and IBS-specific therapies, such as tegaserod (Zelnorm®) and alosetron (Lotronex®). Herbal therapies, including peppermint oil and STW 5, can also reduce IBS.

Where can I learn more about IBS?

Good information about IBS and its treatment can be found at these websites:

- http://familydoctor.org/112.xml
- http://www.aboutibs.org/index.html
- http://digestive.niddk.nih.gov/ddiseases/pubs/ibs/index.htm

---

ment efficacy in this population. Elimination diets and use of probiotics (such as lactobacillus or yogurt) are generally not beneficial.

Ms. Nichols previously showed poor tolerability to treatment with tricyclic antidepressants. She was therefore treated with Lotronex® (alosetron) and pain management skills, including relaxation techniques, coping strategies, and stress management. The psychologist also treated Ms. Nichols for her childhood sexual abuse. She was also provided with an educational flyer (Box 1) to reinforce her treatment recommendations. She reported good symptomatic relief at follow-up in 1 month, which was maintained when she was reassessed 1 year later.

Table 9
Targeted Treatment of Functional Bowel Syndrome

	Nonmedication	Medication
• Restorative treatment	◦ None	◦ None
• Preventive therapies	◦ Cognitive–behavioral therapy ◦ Biofeedback ◦ Pizotifen	◦ Famotidine ◦ Peppermint oil capsules
• Flare techniques	◦ Cognitive–behavioral therapy ◦ Biofeedback	◦ None

2.2. Functional Bowel Syndrome

A recent literature review of the treatment of functional bowel syndrome (recurrent abdominal pain) identified famotidine (Pepcid®), pizotifen (not available in the United States), cognitive–behavioral therapy, biofeedback, and peppermint oil capsules as effective (Table 9) *(26)*. Pain reduction is enhanced by combining medication and nonmedication therapies. A recent study randomized 69 children with recurrent abdominal pain to receive standard medical treatment alone or standard treatment plus five cognitive–behavioral therapy sessions *(27)*. Pain reduction was significantly higher in the combined treatment group for both immediate posttreatment (19% with medical treatment alone versus 22% with combined treatment; $p < 0.05$) and 6 to 12 months after treatment (12 versus 24%; $p < 0.05$).

Ryan's family wanted to focus on herbal and nonmedication treatments to minimize possible treatment side effects. Ryan met with a pain psychologist, who taught stress management, coping techniques, and relaxation skills over six sessions. He also began peppermint oil capsules three times daily. One month later, his episodes of stomachache were occurring infrequently and resolved quickly. Peppermint oil capsules were discontinued and he continued to use his pain management strategies.

3. SUMMARY

Abdominal pain is a common complaint for patients from childhood into later adult life. Patients reporting abdominal pain should be questioned about diet, bowel habits, constitutional symptoms, and family history of GI disease to identify abnormalities suggesting specific pathology. Stomachache is usually nonspecific in children when the pain is peri-umbilical and unrelated to diarrhea, constipation, nausea, weight loss, or fever. Most adults with troublesome chronic abdominal pain will require a sigmoidoscopy or colonoscopy, with additional testing targeted to specific likely clinical scenarios.

REFERENCES

1. Brown J, Berenson K, Cohen P. Documented and self-reported child abuse and adult pain in a community sample. Clin J Pain 2005;21:374–377.
2. Davis DA, Luecken LJ, Zautra AJ. Are reports of childhood abuse related to the experience of chronic pain in adulthood? A meta-analytic review of the literature. Clin J Pain 2005;21:398–405.
3. Drossman DA, Leserman J, Nachman G, et al. Sexual and physical abuse in women with functional or organic gastrointestinal disorders. Ann Intern Med 1990;113:828–833.
4. Thomson H, Francis DM. Abdominal-wall tenderness: a useful sign in the acute abdomen. Lancet 1977;2:1053–1054.
5. Gray DW, Dixon JM, Seabrook G, Collin J. Is abdominal wall tenderness a useful sign in the diagnosis of non-specific abdominal pain? Ann R Coll Surg Engl 1988;70:233–234.
6. Drossman DA, Corazziari E, Talley NJ, Thompson WG, Whitehead WE. Rome II. The Functional Gastrointestinal Disorders. Diagnosis, Pathophysiology and Treatment: A Multinational Consensus. 2nd Ed. McLean, VA: Degnon, 2000.
7. Hungin AS, Whorwell PJ, Tack J, Mearin F. The prevalence, patterns and impact of irritable bowel syndrome: an international survey of 40,000 subjects. Aliment Pharmacol Ther 2003;17:643–650.
8. Moore RA, McQuay HJ. Prevalence of opioid adverse events in chronic nonmalignant pain: systematic review of randomized trials or oral opioids. Arthritis Res Therapy 2005;7:R1046–R1051.
9. Staats PS, Markowitz J, Schein J. Incidence of constipation associated with long-acting opioid therapy: a comparative study. South Med J 2004;97:129–134.
10. McGarrity TJ, Peters DJ, Thompson C, McGarrity SJ. Outcome of patients with chronic abdominal pain referred to chronic pain clinic. Am J Gastroenterol 2000; 95:1812–1816.
11. Petersen Solveig, Bergström, Brulin C. High prevalence of tiredness and pain in young schoolchildren. Scand J Public Health 2003;31:367–374.
12. Chitkara DK, Rawat DJ, Talley NJ. The epidemiology of childhood recurrent abdominal pain in Western countries: a systematic review. Am J Gastroenterol 2005;100:1868–1875.
12a. Alfven G. One hundred cases of recurrent abdominal pain in children: diagnostic procedures and criteria for a psychosomatic diagnosis. Acta Paediatr 2003;92:43–49.
13. Stordal K, Nygaard EA, Bentsen B. Organic abnormalities in recurrent abdominal pain in children. Acta Paediatr 2001;90:638–642.
14. Apley J. The Child With Abdominal Pains. 2nd E d. Oxford, UK: Blackwell Scientific, 1975.
15. American Academy of Pediatrics Subcommittee and NASPGHAN Committee on Chronic Abdominal Pain. Chronic abdominal pain in children: a technical report of the American Academy of Pediatrics and the North American Society for Pediatric Gastroenterology, Hepatology and Nutrition. J Ped Gastroenterol Nutr 2005;40:249–261.

16. American Academy of Pediatrics Subcommittee on Chronic Abdominal Pain and NASPGHAN Committee on Abdominal Pain. Chronic abdominal pain in children: a clinical report of the American Academy of Pediatrics and the North American Society for Pediatric Gastroenterology, Hepatology and Nutrition. J Ped Gastroenterol Nutr 2005;40:245–248.

17. Walker LS, Lipani TA, Greene JW, et al. Recurrent abdominal pain: symptom subtypes based on the Rome II criteria for pediatric functional gastrointestinal disorders. J Ped Gastroenterol Nutr 2004;38:187–191.

18. Platz EA, Willett WC, Colditz GA, et al. Proportion of colon cancer risk that might be preventable in a cohort of middle-aged US men. Cancer Causes Control 2000;11:579–588.

19. Samad AK, Taylor RS, Marshall T, Chapman MA. A meta-analysis of the association of physical activity with reduced risk of colorectal cancer. Colorectal Dis 2005;7:204–213.

20. Larsson SC, Giovannucci E, Bergkvist L, Wolk A. Whole grain consumption and risk of colorectal cancer: a population-based cohort of 60,000 women. Brit J Cancer 2005;92:1803–1807.

21. Bingham SA, Norat T, Moskat A, et al. Is the association with fiber from foods in colorectal cancer confounded by folate intake? Cancer Epidemol Biomarkers Prev 2005;14:1552–1556.

22. Giovannucci E. Diet, body weight, and colorectal cancer: a summary of the epidemiologic evidence. J Womens Health (Larchmt) 2003;12:173–182.

23. Weingarten M, Zalmanovici A, Yaphe J. Dietary calcium supplementation for preventing colorectal cancer and adenomatous polyps. Cochrane Database Syst Rev 2005;3:CD003548.

24. Schoenfeld P. Efficacy of current drug therapies in irritable bowel syndrome: what works and does not work. Gastroenterol Clin N Am 2005;34:319–335.

24a. Holten KB. Irritable bowel syndrome: minimize testing, let symptoms guide treatment. J Fam Pract 2003;52:942–950.

24b. Spanier JA, Howden CW, Jones MP. A systematic review of alternative therapies in the irritable bowel syndrome. Arch Int Med 2003;163:265–274.

25. Madisch A, Holtmann G, Plein K, Hotz J. Treatment of irritable bowel syndrome with herbal preparations: results of a double-blind, randomized, placebo-controlled, multicentre trial. Aliment Pharmacol Ther 2004;19:271–279.

26. Weydert JA, Ball TM, Davis MF. Systemic review of treatment for recurrent abdominal pain. Pediatrics 2003;111:e1–e11.

27. Robins PM, Smith SM, Glutting JJ, Bishop CT. A randomized controlled trial of a cognitive–behavioral family intervention for pediatric recurrent abdominal pain. J Ped Psychol 2005;30:397.

10
Pain in the Whole Body

CHAPTER HIGHLIGHTS

- Patients reporting widespread pain typically endorse high pain severity, disability, and anxiety.
- Common causes of widespread pain include rheumatological conditions, endocrine disorders, infections, and neoplasms.
- Fibromyalgia symptoms improve with long-term treatment.
- Fibromyalgia is best treated with aerobic exercise and pain management skills.
- Arthritis is best treated with exercise, disease-modifying drugs, and symptomatic analgesics.

* * *

This morning, your nurse hands you charts for five new patients. Each patient is a woman complaining of *widespread body pain*, stiffness, and fatigue. In each patient, the pain affects both the left and right sides of the body and is present both above and below the waist. Pain severity is rated between 6 and 8 out of 10 for each patient. Each of these patients was already evaluated by another physician, who diagnosed stress and fibromyalgia in all five. They were all advised that the pain was "nothing to worry about" and to reduce stress and practice distraction techniques. They are seeing you for a second opinion. Here are the stories each patient tells your nurse:

Patient 1: Mrs. Abernathy is a 56-year-old woman who has had generalized pain for the last 6 months. She has been a competitive golfer for the last 15 years. She has barely touched her golf clubs all spring. "I used to go out golfing with the girls every morning. They're so fed up with my whining they stopped calling me. I'd love to get back in the game, but I feel totally fatigued. I have no energy and just want to curl up in bed. All of my muscles and joints just ache."

Patient 2: Ms. Butler is a 48-year-old hospital administrator who used to work out in the gym every morning at 5 AM, work at least 10 hours a day for 6 days each week, and then jog about 5 miles in the evening. For the

From: *Current Clinical Practice: Headache and Chronic Pain Syndromes:*
The Case-Based Guide to Targeted Assessment and Treatment
By: D. A. Marcus © Humana Press, Totowa, NJ

last 2 years, she has been sore and achy all over, and it takes all of her energy to just put in 8 hours at work. "Even talking on the phone worsens my pain! I feel like an old lady who just wants to sit in a rocking chair, knitting. Whenever I tell someone I feel bad, they say, 'But you look great!' If this keeps up, I'm afraid I'll lose my job."

Patient 3: Mrs. Carter is a 67-year-old farmer's wife. "My husband's beginning to slow down too, but we still have our sheep to care for. I always used to help him with chores throughout the day, but now I'm lucky to keep up with the housework. In the past 2 months, I really feel like an old granny. The pain is terrible, and even resting doesn't seem to help. My husband doesn't say anything, but I can tell he's disgusted with me."

Patient 4: Mrs. Daniels is a 45-year-old piano teacher who has had pain for the last 6 months. "I feel so run down and achy. I have pain from my neck to my toes. I really dread having my students come in for lessons. When I grimaced during my last lesson, my student told me, 'Don't worry, Mrs. Daniels. You don't play that badly!'"

Patient 5: Mrs. Everett is a 67-year-old homemaker who complains of having pain for the last 4 months. Her husband has just retired and they had planned to travel, but the pain is holding her back. "I'm just useless. My husband thinks I'm just depressed, but everything gives me pain. It hurts to start moving in the morning and I can't even comb my hair without severe pain. I'm beginning to worry that my marriage will suffer from this darn pain."

1. EVALUATING WIDESPREAD BODY PAIN

Patients with generalized pain complaints are often viewed by health care providers, co-workers, and their families as symptom magnifiers who do not really have pain, but are depressed. A survey of patients with chronic pain with focal or diffuse pain revealed a 17%-higher average pain severity score in those patients with widespread pain, as well as increased prevalence of pain-related disability and anxiety (Fig. 1) *(1)*. Interestingly, despite the common perception that patients with widespread body pain are "just depressed," moderate to severe depression was similar in patients with either diffuse or focal pain. Each of our five patients describes significant impact on daily activities from pain complaints, suggesting high pain severity and disability. These patients also verbalize the typical frustrations and anxieties of patients with widespread pain that sometimes inappropriately shift diagnostic considerations to psychiatric conditions.

Widespread pain is perhaps one of the most challenging chronic pain complaints to evaluate because the causes can include a wide variety of both general medical conditions and chronic pain syndromes (Table 1). Although the

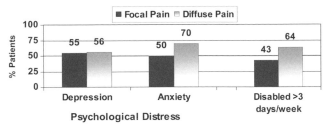

Fig. 1. Differences in disability and emotional distress based on pain distribution. (Based on ref. *1*.)

Table 1
Common Causes of Generalized Pain

Disease category	Specific diseases
• Rheumatology	○ Fibromyalgia ○ Osteoarthritis ○ Rheumatoid arthritis ○ Polymyalgia rheumatica ○ Systemic lupus erythematosus ○ Ankylosing spondylitis ○ Sjögren's syndrome
• Endocrine	○ Hypothyroidism ○ Diabetes ○ Hyperparathyroidism
• Infectious	○ Lyme disease ○ Chronic hepatitis C
• Neoplastic	○ Metastatic cancer ○ Multiple myeloma

chief complaints and brief histories in these five patients are typical, none has provided enough information to formulate an educated diagnosis. Although each patient has the same primary complaint, differences in history and examination can provide ready clues to diagnostic possibilities (Table 2). Extracting these important features depends on a targeted evaluation that focuses on high-yield questions and examination findings that help distinguish among the many possible causes of widespread body pain.

1.1. Developing a High-Yield Targeted Evaluation of Widespread Body Pain

Evaluations of patients with widespread pain should be targeted to specific likely clinical scenarios to help confirm or refute clinical diagnoses. The same

Table 2
Common Chronic Syndromes Causing Widespread Body Pain

	Fibromyalgia	Polymyalgia rheumatica	Osteoarthritis	Rheumatoid arthritis	Hypothyroidism	Lupus
• Age	◦ Any age	◦ >50 years old	◦ Typically >55 years old	◦ Peak onset between ages 35 and 50	◦ Typically >50 years old	◦ Typically in 30s
• Female:male ratio	◦ 6:1	◦ 2:1	◦ 1:1 ◦ Hip > men ◦ Hand and knee > women	◦ 2–3:1	◦ 2–5:1	◦ 9:1
• Pain distribution	◦ Widespread	◦ Proximal shoulder, neck, hip	◦ Asymmetric weight-bearing joints	◦ Symmetric small joints	◦ Generalized aches	◦ Joint and muscle aches
• Associated symptoms	◦ Fatigue ◦ Poor sleep ◦ Numbness ◦ Bowel disturbance	◦ Morning stiffness ◦ Fatigue	◦ Pain worsens with activity and improves with rest ◦ Morning stiffness usually lasts only minutes	◦ Prolonged morning stiffness (>1 hour) ◦ Fatigue	◦ Intolerance to exercise ◦ Poor tolerance to cold ◦ Fatigue	◦ Fatigue ◦ Possibly renal and neurological symptoms
• Constitutional signs	◦ None	◦ Low-grade fever ◦ Weight loss	◦ None	◦ Low-grade fever	◦ Weight gain	◦ Low grade fever ◦ Weight loss
• Physical examination	◦ Normal ROM and neurological and general exams ◦ ≥11 positive tenderpoints	◦ Limited ROM	◦ Limited ROM ◦ Joint crepitus ◦ Bony enlargement	◦ Joint swelling ◦ Restricted ROM	◦ Bradycardia ◦ Sluggish deep tendon reflexes ◦ Muscle weakness ◦ Rash	◦ Puffiness of hands ◦ Symmetric joint swelling
• Laboratory studies	◦ No abnormalities	◦ Elevated inflammatory markers	◦ Bony changes on X-ray	◦ Elevated CRP ◦ Mild anemia ◦ ANA positive in 20 to 30% ◦ X-rays with soft tissue swelling early ◦ Joint changes later	◦ Abnormal thyroid functions ◦ Elevated cholesterol ◦ Mild anemia	◦ Abnormal auto-antibodies (ANA, double-stranded DNA, Sm) and complement levels ◦ Anemia ◦ Leucopenia ◦ Thrombocytopenia

ANA, anti-nuclear antibodies; CRP, C-reactive protein; ROM, range of motion; Sm, Smith monoclonal autoantibodies.

Table 3
Keys to a Targeted Evaluation of Widespread Body Pain

• History	○ Clarify pain location—complete pain drawing
	○ Identify additional medical conditions
	○ Record pain precipitants
	○ Obtain complete review of systems
• Physical examination	○ Vital signs and weight
	○ Musculoskeletal evaluation, including inspection for joint changes and range of motion
	○ Fibromyalgia tenderpoint examination
	○ Neurological examination focusing on strength, reflexes, sensation, and gait testing
• Testing	○ Laboratory testing for blood count, liver enzymes, thyroid function, calcium, and C-reactive protein
	○ Radiographic studies when bony disease is suspected and/or mechanical findings are present

evaluation principles apply to each patient regarding features in the history, physical examination findings, and the need to proceed with testing. Details of the targeted examination are outlined in Table 3. A fibromyalgia tenderpoint examination should be completed for every patient with undiagnosed widespread pain. The fibromyalgia tenderpoint examination is performed by pressing on 18 possible tenderpoints with 4 kg of pressure. Tenderpoint areas are the occiput, trapezius, supraspinatus, gluteal, lower lateral cervical, second costochondral junction, lateral epicondyle, greater trochanter, and medial knee. The examiner presses on each spot with his or her thumb until the nail bed blanches, which is equivalent to about 4 kg of pressure. Patients are asked to rate their pain severity after each spot is pressed on a scale from 0 (*pressure only*) to 10 (*excruciating pain*), and these scores are recorded (Fig. 2). All tenderpoints rated at 2 or higher are considered positive *(2)*. Eleven positive tenderpoints are needed for the diagnosis of fibromyalgia. The number of positive tenderpoints (tenderpoint count) and the total score from all tenderpoints (tenderpoint score) can be used as measures of treatment response in patients diagnosed with fibromyalgia.

1.2. Applying the Targeted Exam to Each Patient

Pain drawings are shown for each patient in Fig. 3. The results of the targeted evaluation and subsequent diagnosis are provided for each patient in Tables 4 to 8. Review the pain drawings, read each patient's findings, decide if additional testing is necessary, and formulate a likely diagnosis. Then read the following sections to compare your interpretations with the patients' diagnoses in the clinic.

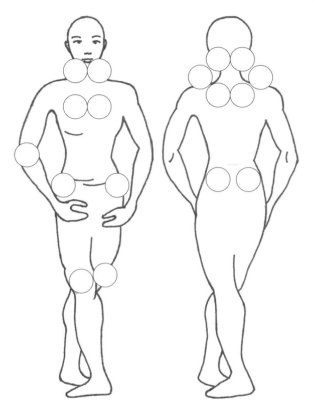

Fig. 2. Recording sheet for fibromyalgia tenderpoint examination. Tenderpoints are shown with circles. Press each possible tenderpoint with the thumb until the nail bed blanches (4 kg of pressure). Record pain score from 0 (pressure only) to 10 (excruciating pain) for each of the 18 tenderpoint areas. (Reprinted with permission from ref. *2a*.)

1.2.1. Patient 1: Mrs. Abernathy—56-Year-Old Golfer (Table 4)

Mrs. Abernathy's history and physical examination suggest possible hypo-thyroidism, which is confirmed with blood work. Mild limitations in active range of motion (ROM) commonly occur in patients with pain complaints resulting from muscle spasm and fear of aggravating pain with movement. More significant ROM restrictions, reproduction of pain with attempted joint movement, and joint crepitus are typically found in patients with mechanical pain or joint pathology. In addition, patients with significant mechanical pain and joint-motion restrictions will usually have the same restriction when the examiner

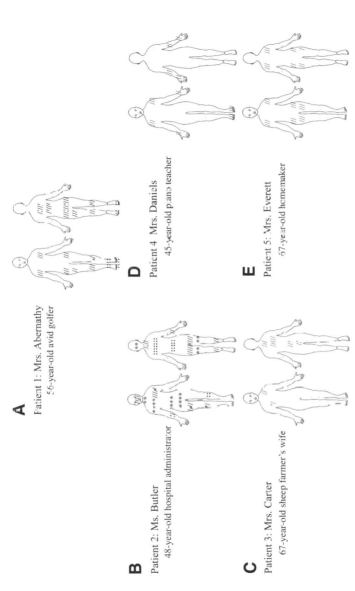

A

Patient 1: Mrs. Abernathy
56-year-old avid golfer

B

Patient 2: Ms. Butler
48-year-old hospital administrator

C

Patient 3: Mrs. Carter
67-year-old sheep farmer's wife

D

Patient 4 Mrs. Daniels
45-year-old piano teacher

E

Patient 5: Mrs. Everett
67-year-old homemaker

Fig. 3. Completed pain drawings for the five patients. (**A**) Patient 1: Mrs. Abernathy—56-year-old avid golfer. (**B**) Patient 2: Ms. Butler—48-year-old hospital administrator. (C) Patient 3: Mrs. Carter—67-year-old sheep farmer's wife. (**D**) Patient 4: Mrs. Daniels—45-year-old piano teacher. (**E**) Patient 5: Mrs. Everett—67-year-old homemaker. Patients are instructed to shade all painful areas using the following key: /// = pain; ::::::: = numbness; **** = burning or hypersensitivity.

171

Table 4
Results of Targeted Evaluation for Patient 1:
Mrs. Abernathy—56-Year-Old Avid Golfer

Targeted assessment	Findings
• History	○ Pain drawing: diffuse pain; numbness in both feet. ○ No additional medical diagnoses. ○ ROS: dry skin, hair loss, feeling cold, constipation, and weight gain. All symptoms new over the last 6 months.
• Physical exam	○ Overweight and apathetic. ○ Mild bradycardia. ○ ROM: neck, back, and limbs mildly limited by pain. ○ 8 Tenderpoints. ○ Normal gait. Mild generalized weakness with no focal neurological deficits.
• Testing	○ Blood work: mild anemia, moderately elevated TSH, and low free T_4; other blood work normal.

ROM, range of motion; ROS, review of systems; TSH, thyroid-stimulating hormone.

asks the patient to move the joint through its range (active ROM), as when the examiner moves the joints while the patient is relaxed (passive ROM). Muscle co-contraction of joint flexors and extensors is common in patients with chronic pain, which significantly reduces active range of motion. When muscle spasm or co-contraction limits active ROM, passive ROM is typically greater. A physical therapy assessment to distinguish restrictions from muscle co-contractions or muscle spasm and mechanical joint disease is sometimes necessary in patients with severe pain complaints who resist testing.

Hypothyroidism is the second most common endocrinological disorder, affecting about 3% of adults *(3,4)*. Like fibromyalgia, hypothyroidism also often includes a wide variety of somatic complaints. Unlike the patient with fibromyalgia who typically has a normal physical examination, the patient with hypothyroidism may display weight gain, dry skin, thinning hair, edema, weakness, and general sluggishness. Generalized aches and pains may also occur in patients with thyroid disease. For example, in a study of subacute thyroiditis, arthralgias or myalgias were present in 16% of patients at presentation *(5)*. Another study of 100 patients with primary hypothyroidism reported joint and/ or muscle pain with stiffness in 19% *(6)*. Hypothyroidism may also result in peripheral neuropathy, evidenced in Mrs. Abernathy by reports of mild numbness in the feet. In early peripheral neuropathy, the general neurological examination is often normal despite reports of sensory disturbance, also as in Mrs. Abernathy.

Table 5
Results of Targeted Evaluation for Patient 2:
Ms. Butler—48-Year-Old Hospital Administrator

Targeted assessment	Findings
• History	○ Pain drawing: diffuse pain, with patchy, nondermatomal numbness and burning.
	○ Pain started after patient was rear-ended with $1000 of damage to her car and no obvious injuries to her other than feeling achy.
	○ No additional medical diagnosis.
	○ ROS: fatigue, poor sleep, eating difficulty with periods of diarrhea and constipation, migraines, frequent episodes of numbness affecting different parts of her body on different days, painful menses, and irritability.
• Physical exam	○ Bright, intelligent, enthusiastic.
	○ Appropriate weight.
	○ Full ROM neck, back, and limbs.
	○ 16 Tenderpoints.
	○ Walks briskly, excellent strength, normal sensation.
• Testing	○ Blood work: normal except for mildly elevated AST.

ROM, range of motion; ROS, review of systems; AST, aspartate aminotransferase.

1.2.2. Patient 2: Ms. Butler—48-Year-Old Hospital Administrator (Table 5)

Ms. Butler's positive review of systems for multisystem complaints, normal physical examination, and relatively normal blood work are consistent with a diagnosis of fibromyalgia. Her elevated aspartate aminotransferase is probably a reflection of alcohol with last night's dinner.

Ms. Butler is a very typical fibromyalgia patient—bright, hardworking, and motivated. Like Ms. Butler, patients with fibromyalgia often look vigorous and energetic despite complaints of high fatigue. Patients with fibromyalgia often hear that they look great and have excellent musculoskeletal and neurological examinations: "You look too good and move too well to have so much pain!" Laboratory testing is also typically normal. It is important to remember, however, that fibromyalgia is not a diagnosis of exclusion. Diagnosis requires widespread pain and the presence of at least 11 positive tenderpoints. Fibromyalgia should be considered in patients with widespread pain, numerous somatic complaints, no obvious medical conditions, and normal medical, neurological, and musculoskeletal examinations.

Fibromyalgia may occur after trauma or spontaneously. The etiology of its symptoms is unknown. Fibromyalgia affects about 3% of women and 0.5% of men *(7)*. Although fibromyalgia is often perceived as a disease of young

Table 6
Results of Targeted Evaluation for Patient 3:
Mrs. Carter—67-Year-Old Farmer's Wife

Targeted assessment	Findings
• History	○ Pain drawing: pain spine and ribs; worst pain is in her back. ○ Only other medical problem is hypertension. ○ ROS: 10-pound unintentional, but welcome, weight loss, as well as fatigue and shortness of breath. She has also been treated for an upper respiratory infection and two urinary tract infections in the last several months, which is unusual for her.
• Physical exam	○ Sluggish, slow moving, overweight woman ○ Mild pedal edema. ○ Tenderness over her spine and low back. ○ Four tenderpoints. ○ Normal neurological exam
• Testing	○ Blood work: anemia, mildly elevated creatinine, and hypercalcemia

ROM, range of motion; ROS, review of systems.

women, its prevalence rises with increasing age, affecting 7% of women 60 years of age and older.

1.2.3. Patient 3: Mrs. Carter—67-Year-Old Farmer's Wife (Table 6)

Location of pain over the spine and ribs and an elevated serum calcium suggest bony disease is the cause of Mrs. Carter's pain. Serum and urine electrophoresis identify monoclonal protein, confirming the clinical diagnosis of multiple myeloma (MM).

In 2005, an estimated 16,000 people were diagnosed with MM in the United States, making it the second most common hematological cancer after non-Hodgkin's lymphoma *(8)*. MM also ranks among the top 10 cancers resulting in death in women. The risk for MM increases with certain occupations, including precision printing occupations (odds ratio [OR] = 10.1), pharmacists/dieticians/therapists (OR = 6.1), heating equipment operators (OR = 4.7), roofers (OR = 3.3), hand molders/casters (OR = 3.0), and, as in the case of Mrs. Carter, sheep farmers (OR = 1.7) *(9)*. Obesity, lower socioeconomic status, and African-American race also increase risk *(10)*.

1.2.4. Patient 4: Mrs. Daniels—45-Year-Old Piano Teacher (Table 7)

Mrs. Daniels' blood work suggests an inflammatory condition. History of breast cancer warranted a bone scan, which was negative for metastatic disease. Rheumatoid arthritis (RA) is distinguished from osteoarthritis (OA) by

Table 7
Results of Targeted Evaluation for Patient 4:
Mrs. Daniels—45-Year-Old Piano Teacher

Targeted assessment	Findings
• History	○ Pain drawing: pain over joints in both shoulders, elbows, hands, and feet. Her worst pain is in her hands, which is limiting her ability to play the piano.
	○ Pain began slowly over about 6 weeks without injury. She first noticed stiffness in a couple of her fingers that seemed to worsen when she tried to move them. Since then, the pain and stiffness seem to come and go.
	○ Morning stiffness generally lasts for 2 to 3 hours, causing her to discontinue morning lessons.
	○ Treated for breast cancer with lumpectomy and radiation 4 years ago. Negative mammograms since.
	○ ROS: fatigue and occasional low-grade fevers; weight stable.
• Physical exam	○ Normal vital signs and weight.
	○ Swelling and tenderness in the metacarpophalangeal joints in both hands.
	○ Restricted ROM in hands and shoulders.
	○ Nine tenderpoints.
	○ Normal neurological exam.
• Testing	○ Blood work: mild anemia, positive ANA, and elevated C-reactive protein.

ROM, range of motion; ROS, review of systems; ANA, anti-nuclear antibodies.

the location of joint symptoms. As in Mrs. Daniels, RA usually has symmetrical involvement of small joints, whereas OA has asymmetrical involvement of large, weight-bearing joints. History of symmetrical, distal joint involvement and blood work consistent with an inflammatory arthritis warranted testing for rheumatoid factor (RF) auto-antibody, X-rays of the hands and feet, and a synovial fluid analysis. RF was positive, as is seen in 60 to 80% of patients with RA *(11)*. Disease specificity of RF auto-antibody for RA, however, is low (66%). A variety of other rheumatological conditions, including OA, may also be associated with a positive RF. Therefore, RF testing should not be used as a general screening tool in patients with widespread pain. In addition, RF titers may be low in early RA. As was seen in Mrs. Daniels, X-rays of early RA are often only remarkable for soft-tissue swelling; however, bony erosions develop rapidly with active disease during the first 2 years. Synovial fluid analysis failed to identify any other causes of inflammatory arthritis, such as gout or infectious arthritis.

RA affects about 0.5 to 1% of adults *(12)*. Morning stiffness and joint swelling are characteristics features of RA. Although most arthritic patients report

Table 8
Results of Targeted Evaluation for Patient 5:
Mrs. Schmidt—67-Year-Old Homemaker

Targeted assessment	Findings
• History	○ Pain drawing: symmetrical pain in the shoulders, hips, and thighs. The worst pain is in the shoulders.
	○ She is very stiff for about 1 hour in the morning, and trying to move the joints intensifies the pain. She is having trouble getting out of bed and has started asking her husband to comb her hair in the mornings.
	○ No other medical conditions.
	○ ROS: low-grade fevers, fatigue, loss of appetite, and weight loss.
• Physical exam	○ Temperature 99°F.
	○ Restricted ROM in the shoulders.
	○ Muscle tenderness to palpation.
	○ Seven tenderpoints.
• Testing	○ Blood work: normal except for elevated C-reactive protein

ROM, range of motion; ROS, review of systems.

stiffness after extended rest, this stiffness generally improves fairly rapidly after the joints have been moved for patients with OA. As reported by Mrs. Daniels, morning stiffness is often pronounced and persists for longer than 1 hour in RA.

1.2.5. Patient 5: Mrs. Everett—67-Year-Old Homemaker (Table 8)

Mrs. Everett's age, pain distribution, and elevated C-reactive protein (CRP) suggest the diagnosis of polymyalgia rheumatica (PMR). Formal diagnostic criteria for PMR typically require an erythrocyte sedimentation rate (ESR) greater than 40 mm/hour *(9)*. CRP, however, is a more sensitive measure for both diagnosis and determination of disease activity *(13)*. In a large survey of 177 patients diagnosed with PMR, ESR was less than or equal to 30 mm/hour in 10 patients (6%). CRP was only falsely negative in two patients (1%). In addition, only one of the patients with a negative ESR also had a negative CRP.

PMR is characterized by bilateral proximal pain and stiffness in the shoulders and hips. PMR occurs in older patients, peaking in incidence between 70 and 80 years old *(14)*. The most common complaint is difficulty combing the hair. Other typical complaints include difficulty getting out of bed or rising from a chair, especially after prolonged sitting.

2. TREATING CHRONIC WIDESPREAD BODY PAIN

Disease-specific restorative treatments are available for many medical conditions. For example, PMR, MM, and hypothyroidism may be treated with spe-

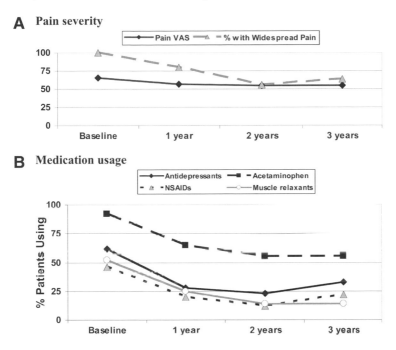

Fig. 4. Long-term outcome with standard fibromyalgia treatment. (A) Pain severity. (B) Medication usage. (Based on ref. *15*.) NSAIDs, nonsteroidal anti-inflammatory drugs; VAS, visual analog scale (0 = *no pain*, 100 = *excruciating pain*).

cific disease-targeted treatments. Hypothyroidism was corrected in Mrs. Abernathy with thyroid hormone supplementation. Mrs. Carter was treated with melphalan and prednisone for MM, with long acting opioids added for pain control. Mrs. Everett experienced rapid symptomatic relief after treatment with prednisone for PMR. Treating fibromyalgia in Ms. Butler and RA in Mrs. Daniels requires long-term chronic pain management.

2.1. Fibromyalgia

Although there are no curative treatments for fibromyalgia, most patients with fibromyalgia experience significant improvement with treatment. A longitudinal study following 59 patients with fibromyalgia who were treated in university and community practices for 3 years identified significant reductions in pain and medication use *(15)*. Pain scores were significantly decreased after 1 year ($p < 0.05$) and continued to be significantly decreased for the full 3 years ($p < 0.01$; Fig. 4A). The average number of positive tenderpoints (tenderpoint count) also

Table 9
Targeted Treatment of Fibromyalgia

	Nonmedication	Medication
• Restorative treatment	○ Possibly aerobic exercise	○ None
• Preventive therapies	○ Aerobic exercise ○ Stress management, relaxation, cognitive restructuring ○ Pacing skills, body mechanics	○ Antidepressants
• Flare techniques	○ Relaxation ○ Stretching exercises for additional myofascial pain	○ Tramadol

decreased significantly from 14 at baseline to 11 after 1 year and 10 after 3 years ($p < 0.001$). Use of antidepressants, nonsteroidal anti-inflammatory drugs (NSAIDs), and muscle relaxants was also significantly decreased at each assessment point ($p < 0.05$; Fig. 4B). A follow-up study including 70 patients followed for 3 years showed moderate to marked improvement in 47% *(16)*.

There are no clearly restorative treatments for fibromyalgia. The most effective treatments include aerobic exercise, education, and psychological pain management techniques (Table 9). The most effective class of medications for fibromyalgia is the antidepressants, although only about one-third of patients with fibromyalgia improve with antidepressants *(17)*. Antidepressants are perhaps most beneficial in patients with fibromyalgia who have additional somatic complaints, including sleep disturbance, depression, frequent headache, and/ or irritable bowel syndrome. A 450-mg daily dose of pregabalin was recently shown to significantly reduce fibromyalgia symptoms in comparison with placebo, although pain reduction was modest *(18)*. Mean reduction in an 11-point pain severity scale was only 0.9.

Flare techniques should also focus on nonmedication therapies. NSAIDs are typically no more effective than placebo for fibromyalgia *(17)*. Combination therapy with 37.5 mg tramadol plus 325 mg acetaminophen (one to two tablets per dose) taken four times daily is superior to placebo *(19)*.

Ms. Butler was given an educational flyer describing fibromyalgia (Box 1). She was also prescribed an aerobic exercise program, which included her choice of a gradually increasing walking or swimming program that increased by walking one-half mile or swimming four laps per week. The office nurse provided sleep hygiene information, with Ms. Butler planning to avoid taking work to bed at night and drinking caffeinated beverages after dinner. Before retiring, she will take a brisk walk, followed by neck stretches and deep breathing. Ms. Butler also worked with a psychologist to learn relaxation tech-

---

Box 1
Educational Flyer for Patients With Fibromyalgia

What is fibromyalgia?

Fibromyalgia affects about 2% of adults, more often women than men. Fibromyalgia is a condition causing increased sensitivity to pain. Patients with fibromyalgia have pain in many different parts of their bodies and often notice that they are especially sensitive to pressure and touch. In addition to feeling pain, patients with fibromyalgia often have a variety of other symptoms, including fatigue, sleep disturbance, stiffness, numbness, bowel and bladder complaints, depression, and anxiety. Fibromyalgia symptoms do *not* progress to cause severe weakness, paralysis, or the inability to move or walk.

Although patients with fibromyalgia experience many unpleasant symptoms, they often hear their doctors tell them, "But you look terrific," and "All of your tests are normal." This does not mean that fibromyalgia is imaginary. Doctors just have not figured out what causes fibromyalgia. So far, research shows that fibromyalgia does not seem to be caused by infections, genetic defects, or exposures in the environment.

How is fibromyalgia treated?

Although medical science has not found the cause for fibromyalgia, the good news is that there are many treatments that help reduce fibromyalgia symptoms. About half of those patients with fibromyalgia will report that their symptoms are much or very much better after a couple of years, so there is a light at the end of the tunnel.

First, your doctor will need to make sure that your symptoms are not caused by other treatable medical conditions. Once your doctor has diagnosed you with fibromyalgia, ask about beginning an exercise program. Aerobic exercise is one of the most effective treatments for reducing fibromyalgia symptoms.

Other effective treatments include physical therapy, occupational therapy to help teach pacing skills and the appropriate use of body mechanics, and pain management skills, such as stress management, relaxation, and coping skills. Medications are only modestly helpful for fibromyalgia. Antidepressants are the most helpful group of medications and work best if you also have problems with your sleep, digestive system, and/or mood as part of your fibromyalgia symptoms. Most pain killers are not very helpful for fibromyalgia.

Where can I learn more?

Good information about the diagnosis and treatment of fibromyalgia can be found at these websites:

- http://familydoctor.org
- http://fmaware.org
- http://fmpartnership.org
- http://www.hopkins-arthritis.som.jhmi.edu/other/fibromyalgia.html

Table 10
Targeted Treatment of Arthritis

	Nonmedication	Medication

• Restorative treatment	○ Possibly aerobic exercise	○ DMARDs for RA
		  ▪ Sulfasalazine
		  ▪ Hydroxychloroquine
		  ▪ Methotrexate for advanced RA (Second-line: tumor necrosis factor-α or interleukin-1 inhibitors)

• Preventive therapies	○ ROM, strengthening, and aerobic exercise
	○ Aquatherapy
	○ Stress management, relaxation, cognitive restructuring
	○ Pacing skills, body mechanics
	○ Obesity reduction
		○ DMARDs for RA
		  ▪ Sulfasalazine
		  ▪ Hydroxychloroquine
		  ▪ Methotrexate for advanced RA (Second-line: tumor necrosis factor-α or interleukin-1 inhibitors)

• Flare techniques	○ Relaxation ○ Stretching exercises for additional myofascial pain	○ Acetaminophen for OA ○ NSAIDs for RA

DMARDs, disease-modifying anti-rheumatic drugs; NSAIDs, nonsteroidal anti-inflammatory drugs; OA, osteoarthritis; RA, rheumatoid arthritis; ROM, range of motion.

niques and coping skills. They also discussed more realistic scheduling of her day to develop appropriate expectations for the amount of tasks she can reasonably manage. Finally, she worked with an occupational therapist who further addressed appropriate pacing of both work and household tasks. She was advised to change her work desk so she could maintain better posture on the job, and she started using a telephone headset instead of holding a handheld phone between her cheek and shoulder so her pain would not flare when frequently talking on the phone.

2.2. Treating Arthritis

Arthritis treatment differs for patients with degenerative versus inflammatory arthritis (Table 10). Nonmedication and medication treatments help both inflammatory and non-inflammatory arthritis. Although joint stiffness may encourage patients to decrease exercise and activity levels, both strengthening and aerobic exercise significantly reduce pain and disability in patients with OA or RA (20,21). An interesting recent study showed that biweekly, high-intensity exercise was actually associated with less long-term joint damage than physical therapy alone in RA (22). During a 2-year observation, relevant radiographic progression of joint damage was observed in 11% of patients treated with exercise versus 22% treated with physical therapy ($p < 0.05$).

Despite these clear benefits from exercise, a recent large survey of more than 56,000 patients with physician-diagnosed arthritis found that only 42% had ever been advised to exercise to improve arthritis symptoms *(23)*. Obesity reduction is also important because obesity has been linked to the development of OA in the hands, hips, and knees *(24)*.

There are no restorative or preventive medications for OA. OA pain may be treated with analgesics. There is no additional analgesic benefit from an antiinflammatory analgesic compared with acetaminophen.

Disease-modifying anti-rheumatic drugs are first-line treatment for RA because they retard bony destruction and preserve function when used in early disease *(25)*. Radiographic studies also document bone repair with long-term use of disease-modifying anti-rheumatic drugs *(26)*. NSAIDs provide good symptomatic relief in RA, although they do not impede joint destruction.

Ms. Daniels was provided with an educational flyer (Box 2) and treated with sulfasalazine, which offers faster relief and better retardation of bony destruction than hydroxychloroquine. She was also prescribed naproxen (Naprosyn®)twice daily for symptomatic relief. Ms. Daniels started biweekly exercise after using an Internet site (http://www.arthritis.org/events/getinvolved/ProgramsServices/default.asp) to locate a nearby facility trained to administer the Arthritis Foundation Aquatic Program and People with Arthritis Can Exercise classes her doctor recommended. She adjusted her piano appointments to later in the day to avoid lessons during her early-morning stiffness, and was delighted when one of her students exclaimed, "Ms. Daniels! You finally learned to play the piano yourself!"

3. SUMMARY

Remember that widespread body pain can be caused by a variety of conditions. Do not be dissuaded from carefully evaluating diffuse body aches and pain because reported pain levels, associated disability, and anxiety seem excessively high. Diffuse pain may be the presenting complaint for a wide variety of medical conditions. In addition, patients with widespread chronic pain syndromes tend to have more disability and distress than patients with focal pain *(1)*. These patients typically require a more in-depth evaluation and aggressive treatment.

REFERENCES

1. Marcus DA. Headache and other types of chronic pain. Headache 2003;43:49–53.
2. Okifuji A, Turk DC, Sinclair JD, Starz TW, Marcus DA. A standardized manual tender point survey. I. Development and determination of a threshold point for the identification of positive tender points in fibromyalgia syndrome. J Rheumatol 1997;24:377–383.

Box 2
Educational Flyer for Patients With Arthritis

What is arthritis?

Arthritis is a common cause of joint pain affecting about 15% of adults. The two most common types of arthritis are osteoarthritis (OA) and rheumatoid arthritis (RA). OA is caused by wear and tear on the joints. With overuse, joints can develop calcium deposits and the cartilage between the bones may begin to wear down or erode. OA typically affects those joints that get the most use—the neck, back, hips, and knees. OA pain typically worsens with activity and improves with rest. Morning stiffness usually goes away after moving around for a few minutes.

RA is caused by inflammation or swelling around the joints. RA typically affects the shoulders, elbows, hands, knees, and feet. The joints often become deformed in patients with RA. Joints are often very stiff in the morning, with stiffness usually lasting more than 1 hour. Patients with RA often have other symptoms besides pain, including low-grade fevers and fatigue. The lungs, heart, and nervous systems may also become affected with RA.

How is arthritis treated?

Both OA and RA are treated with reduction in obesity and exercise. Physical therapy stretching exercises, aerobic exercise, and aqua or pool therapy help improve arthritis. Be sure to talk to your doctor or physical therapist before starting any new exercise program. Your doctor may also recommend that you work with an occupational therapist to help modify your activities so you can do more at work and at home with less pain.

OA is not caused by inflammation, so pain is usually treated with acetaminophen. Anti-inflammatory medications generally provide no additional pain relief for OA.

RA is treated with anti-inflammatory medications and medications designed to prevent bony deformities, called disease-modifying anti-rheumatic drugs.

Pain management skills, such as stress management, relaxation, techniques, and developing coping skills also help decrease arthritis pain.

Where can I learn more about arthritis?

Good information about the diagnosis and treatment of arthritis can be found at these websites:

- http://familydoctor.org
- http://www.hopkins-arthritis.org
- http://www.arthritis.org/AFStore/StartRead.asp?idProduct=3359
- http://www.arthritis.org.sg/101/treat/exercise.html

2a. Marcus DA. Chronic Pain: A Primary Care Guide to Practical Management. Totowa, NJ: Humana Press, 2005.

3. Bjøro T, Holmen J, Krüger Ø, et al. Prevalence of thyroid disease, thyroid dysfunction and thyroid peroxidase antibodies in a large, unselected population. The Health Study of Nord-Trøndelag (HUNT). Eur J Endocrinol 2000;143:639–647.

4. Flynn RV, MacDonald TM, Morris AD, Jung RT, Leese GP. The thyroid epidemiology, audit, and research study: thyroid dysfunction in the general population. J Clin Endocrinol Metab 2004;89:3879–3884.

5. Fatourechi V, Aniszewski JP, Fatourechi GZ, Atkinson EJ, Jacobsen SJ. Clinical features and outcome of subacute thyroiditis in an incidence cohort: Olmstead County, Minnesota, study. J Clin Endocrinol Metab 2003;88:2100–2105.

6. Carette S, Lefrancois L. Fibrositis and primary hypothyroidism. J Rheumatol 1988;15:1418–1421.

7. Wolfe F, Ross K, Anderson J, Russell IJ, Hebert L. The prevalence and characteristics of fibromyalgia in the general population. Arthritis Rheum 1995;8:19–28.

8. Jemal A, Murray T, Ward E, et al. Cancer statistics, 2005. CA Cancer J Clin 2005; 55:10–30.

9. Baris D, Silverman DT, Brown LM, et al. Occupation, pesticide exposure and risk of multiple myeloma. Scand J Work Environ Health 2004;30:215–222.

10. Benjamin M, Reddy S, Brawley OW. Myeloma and race: a review of the literature. Cancer Metastasis Rev 2003;22:87–93.

11. Steiner G, Smolen J. Autoantibodies in rheumatoid arthritis and their clinical significance. Arthritis Res 2002;4(Suppl 2):S1–S5.

12. Alamanos Y, Drosos AA. Epidemiology of adult rheumatoid arthritis. Autoimmun Rev 2005;4:130–136.

13. Cantini F, Salvarani C, Olivieri I, et al. Erythrocyte sedimentation rate and c-reactive protein in the evaluation of disease activity and severity in polymyalgia rheumatica: a prospective follow-up study. Semin Arthritis Rheum 2000;30:17–24.

14. Salvarani C, Cantini F, Boiardi L, Hunder GG. Polymyalgia rheumatica. Best Pract Res Clin Rheumatology 2004;18:705–722.

15. Pöyhiä R, Da Costa D, Fitzcharles M. Pain and pain relief in fibromyalgia patients followed for three years. Arthritis Care Res 2001;45:355–361.

16. Fitzcharles MA, Costa DD, Pöyhiä R. A study of standard care in fibromyalgia syndrome: a favorable outcome. J Rheumatol 2003;30:154–159.

17. Lautenschläger J. Present state of medication therapy in fibromyalgia syndrome. Scand J Rheumatol Suppl 2000;113:32–36.

18. Crofford LJ, Rowbotham MC, Mease PJ, et al. Pregabalin for the treatment of fibromyalgia syndrome: results of a randomized, double-blind, placebo-controlled trial. Arthritis Rheum 2005;52:1264–1273.

19. Bennett RM, Kamin M, Kamin R, Rosenthal N. Tramadol and acetaminophen combination tablets in the treatment of fibromyalgia pain: a double-blind, randomized, placebo-controlled study. Am J Med 2003;114:537–545.

20. Roddy E, Zhang W, Doherty M. Aerobic walking or strengthening exercise for osteoarthritis of the knee? A systematic review. Ann Rheum Dis 2005;64: 544–548.

21. De Jong Z, Munneke M, Zwinderman AH, et al. Is a long-term high-intensity exercise program effective and safe in patients with rheumatoid arthritis? Arthritis Rheum 2003;48:2415–2424.

22. Maxwell L, Tugwell P. High–intensity exercise for rheumatoid arthritis was associated with less joint damage of the hands and feet than physical therapy. ACP J Club 2005;142:73.
23. Fontaine KR, Bartlett SJ, Heo M. Are health care professionals advising adults with arthritis to become more physically active? Arthritis Rheum 2005;53: 279–283.
24. Oliveria SA, Felson DT, Cirillo PA, Reed JI, Walker AM. Body weight, body mass index, and incident symptomatic osteoarthritis of the hand, hip, and knee. Epidemiology 1999;10:161–166.
25. Sokka T, Möttönen T, Hannonen P. Disease-modifying anti-rheumatic drug use according to the "sawtooth" treatment strategy improves the functional outcome in rheumatoid arthritis: results of a long-term follow-up study with review of the literature. Rheumatology 2000;39:34–42.
26. Rau R, Herborn G. Healing phenomena of erosive changes in rheumatoid arthritis patients undergoing disease-modifying antirheumatic drug therapy. Arthritis Rheum 1996;39:162–168.

11

General Chronic Pain Management Techniques

CHAPTER HIGHLIGHTS

- Chronic pain is usually best managed with the combination of medication and nonmedication techniques.
- Medication treatment should focus on pain prevention therapies, rather than flare treatment.
- Effective nonmedication techniques include exercise, instruction in pacing and body mechanics, relaxation training, and stress management.
- Healthy lifestyle changes improve general health and decrease pain complaints.

* * *

For most patients with chronic pain, pain will persist for many months or years, and no treatment will be available to cure their pain. For this reason, the patient must become an active participant in the treatment team. Therapy should focus on self-management, rather than passive therapies performed on the patient. Self-management allows the patient to initially receive medical therapy, but then reduce the number of doctor and therapy visits as skills are learned and integrated into a home routine. In this way, patient identity can shift from "Mrs. Smith—patient with chronic pain," whose day revolves around going to medical appointments, to "Mrs. Smith—first grade teacher," who happens to do a relaxation and exercise program twice daily for pain management and, occasionally, has adjustments to her pain program through medical visits.

The doctor reinforces self-management by instructing patients in the proper use of medications for daily prevention and flares, rather than asking the patient to report to the clinic for an injection or evaluation whenever a pain flare occurs. The physical therapist focuses on self-management by teaching the patient skills he or she can use regularly on his or her own to reduce daily pain and pain flares rather than performing passive, in-office treatments, such as massage and other soothing modalities. Passive therapy may be included when treatment is initiated to decrease pain to more tolerable levels that allow patient participation in active exercise. Other passive

From: *Current Clinical Practice: Headache and Chronic Pain Syndromes:*
The Case-Based Guide to Targeted Assessment and Treatment
By: D. A. Marcus © Humana Press, Totowa, NJ

therapies, such as chiropractics and acupuncture, are similarly often beneficial for treating acute pain, but show little long-term benefit for chronic pain, and reinforce continued reliance on health care providers.

1. MEDICATIONS

Medications may be divided into preventive and flare management therapies. For most types of chronic pain, treatment should focus on pain-preventive techniques designed to reduce both daily pain severity and the frequency of pain flares. Preventive therapy is more likely to reduce overall disability compared with flare treatment.

A large, systematic review of outpatient chronic pain management analyzed data from the existing literature to identify the number of patients needed to be treated (NNT) to achieve an effective response for an assortment of medication therapies (Table 1) *(1)*. None of these individual therapies was effective for most patients. These data show that a variety of therapies may be effective for chronic pain, but the individual patient will probably need to try several therapies before finding one that works well for him or her.

1.1. Preventive Therapy

Prevention therapy that targets specific pain syndromes is typically more effective than nonspecific treatment with analgesics (Table 2). Neuropathic pain, headaches, and fibromyalgia may benefit from treatment with antidepressants or some anti-epileptics. Selection of an antidepressant depends on associated comorbid conditions (Table 3). In general, tricyclic antidepressants are the most effective group of antidepressants for analgesic benefit. Other antidepressants, such as the selective serotonin reuptake inhibitors (SSRIs), selective noradrenaline reuptake inhibitors (SNRIs), and the noradrenaline and dopamine uptake inhibitor bupropion, may be used as second-line therapy in patients who are unable to tolerate tricyclics. Animal studies show analgesic effects from SSRIs resulting from effects on both opioid receptors and serotonergic mechanisms *(2)*. Clinical efficacy for pain reduction with both neuropathic pain and chronic headache, however, is inferior with SSRIs and SNRIs compared with tricyclics *(3,4)*.

1.2. Flare Management

Flare management therapies should be reserved for infrequent, severe flares that are expected to be long-lasting (Table 4). Frequent pain flares that occur throughout the day or brief flares typically lasting a few hours are usually well managed with nonmedication techniques, such as stretching, ice, heat, and relaxation. In general, patients should be advised to limit the use of flare medications to 2 days or less per week. More frequent use suggests a need to increase prevention therapy.

Table 1
Number Needed to Treat for Efficacy for Pain Medications

Medication	NNT	Medication	NNT
• Minor analgesics		• Topical NSAIDs	3.0
○ Acetaminophen	2.9	• Topical capsaicin	3.9
○ Ibuprofen	2.0	• Antipdepressants	3.0
○ Tramadol	8.2	• Anti-epileptics	2.5
○ Propoxyphene	7.5		

NNT, number needed to treat; NSAIDs, nonsteroidal anti-inflammatory drugs. (Based on ref. *1*.)

Table 2
Preventive Medications

Drug class	Conditions treated	Examples
• Antidepressants	○ Neuropathy ○ Headache ○ Fibromyalgia ○ Depression ○ Anxiety ○ Sleep disturbance	○ Tricyclics ▪ amitriptyline (Elavil®) ▪ impiramine (Tofranil®) ○ SSRIs ▪ paroxetine (Paxil®) ○ SNRIs ▪ venlafaxine (Effexor®) ▪ buproprion (Wellbutrin®)
• Anti epileptics	○ Neuropathy ○ Headache ○ Anxiety ▪ gabapentin ○ Sleep disturbance ▪ gabapentin	○ Gabapentin ▪ Neurontin® ○ Pregabalin ▪ Lycira® ○ Lamotrigine ▪ Lamictal® ○ Topiramate ▪ Topamax®
• Analgesics	○ Disabling, nonresponsive pain	○ Long-acting opioids ▪ morphine (MS Contin®, Kadian®) ▪ methadone ▪ fentanyl (Duragesic®) ▪ oxycodone (Oxycontin®)

SNRI, selective noradrenaline reuptake inhibitor; SSRI, selective serotonin reuptake inhibitor.

Opioids provide stronger analgesic potency for non-inflammatory pain, without risk from prostaglandin-related effects. However, about 30% of primary care patients prescribed opioids for chronic pain demonstrate medication misuse or abuse, including reporting lost/stolen prescriptions, obtaining opioids from secondary sources, and repeatedly requesting early refills *(5)*.

Table 3
Antidepressant Guide

Antidepressant	Comorbid condition
• Imipramine (Tofranil®) • Paroxetine (Paxil®)	○ Anxiety
• Amitriptyline (Elavil®) • Sinequan (Doxepin®)	○ Sleep disturbance
• Nortriptyline (Pamelor®) • Protryptyline (Vivactil®)	○ No sleep disturbance
• Paroxetine (Paxil®) • Venlafaxine (Effexor®) • Bupropion (Wellbutrin®)	○ Poor tolerability of tricyclics

Select antidepressant based on comorbid conditions.

Table 4
Flare Management Medications

Drug class	Conditions treated	Examples
• Nonopioid analgesics	○ Degenerative arthritis ○ Non-inflammatory pain flares	○ Acetaminophen ○ Tramadol ▪ Ultram®

• Anti-inflammatory
analgesics
	○ Inflammatory arthritis
	○ Headache/migraine
		○ Aspirin
		○ NSAIDs
		  ▪ ibuprofen (Motrin®)
		  ▪ naproxen (Naprosyn®/Aleve®)

• Short-acting
opioids
	○ Disabling, nonrespon-
	sive pain flares
		○ Hydrocodone
		  ▪ Vicodin®
		○ Oxycodone
		  ▪ Percocet®

• Triptans	○ Migraine	○ Sumatriptan
		  ▪ Imitrex®
		○ rizatriptan
		  ▪ Maxalt®
		○ eletriptan
		  ▪ Relpax®
		○ zolmitriptan
		  ▪ Zomig®
		○ almotriptan
		  ▪ Axert®
		○ naratriptan
		  ▪ Amerge®
		○ frovatriptan
		  ▪ Frova®

NSAID, nonsteroidal anti-inflammatory drug.

Table 5
Pain Medications During Pregnancy and Attempted Conception

| | FDA risk category | | |
	A or B	C	D or X
	Safe	Use if benefit > risk	Avoid
• Prevention	∘ β-Blockers	∘ Tricyclic	∘ Valproate
	∘ SSRI antidepressants	antidepressants	
	∘ Buproprion	∘ Venlafaxine	
	∘ Long-acting opioids[a]	∘ Gabapentin	
		∘ Topiramate	
		∘ Lamotrigine	
• Flare	∘ Acetaminophen	∘ Triptan	∘ Aspirin
	∘ NSAIDs first and		∘ NSAIDs third
	second trimesters		trimester
	∘ Opioids[a]		∘ Ergotamine

[a] Long-acting oxycodone is FDA category B, whereas other short- and long-acting opioids are category C. Clinical experience, however, suggests safe short-term use with pregnancy.

NSAIDs, nonsteroidal anti-inflammatory drugs; SSRIs, selective serotonin reuptake inhibitors.

Patients prescribed opioids, therefore, need chart documentation stating the reason(s) for selecting an opioid, such as failure or intolerability of other analgesics. Furthermore, monitors for compliance, such as random urine screens and careful documentation of prescriptions, should also be routinely used.

1.3. Pain Medications During Pregnancy

The selection of medications prescribed to women capable of child-bearing is influenced by medication safety during pregnancy (Table 5). Gabapentin may be used during attempted conception and early pregnancy. Because gabapentin may adversely affect development of the fetal bony growth plate, it should be discontinued as pregnancy progresses. Opioids are best limited to infrequent, intermittent use. Patients who have been chronically using daily opioids during mid-to-late pregnancy must continue daily opioids because of the risks of fetal mortality and premature labor associated with intrauterine fetal opioid withdrawal *(6)*.

2. HERBS, MINERALS, AND VITAMINS

Few well-controlled studies have shown benefit from herbal, mineral, or vitamin therapy in chronically painful conditions, with the exception of migraine. Externally applied capsaicin is well established as an effective therapy for neuralgia and arthritis pain. A recent small, open-label study compared pain reduction in patients with fibromyalgia and osteoarthritis with a combination of reduced iso-α-acids from hops, rosemary extract, and oleanic acid (Meta050). Pain reduction after 8 weeks was significant in osteoarthritis (50%; $p < 0.0001$), but not fibromyalgia (25%) *(7)*. In addition, insomnia may be treated with valerian, whereas depression may be treated with St. John's wort.

A variety of natural therapies have demonstrated efficacy for reducing migraine frequency in placebo-controlled trials *(8)*:

* 600 mg of magnesium daily.
* 400 mg of riboflavin daily.
* 150 mg of coenzyme Q10 daily.
* 100 mg of 0.2% feverfew daily.
* 50 to 100 mg of butterbur twice daily.

These therapies should not be used during pregnancy. Magnesium and butterbur are also helpful in children with migraine *(8)*. Peppermint oil effectively treats tension-type headaches, but has not been tested in migraine *(9)*. Recently, a single open-label study reported reduction in migraine frequency by 61% and severity by 51% with 3 mg of melatonin at bedtime *(10)*. Controlled studies with melatonin as a migraine therapy are not available.

3. NONMEDICATION TREATMENT

Combining nonmedication with medication treatments results in benefits greater than using either treatment alone *(11,12)*. Nonmedication treatments offer patients successful techniques to improve daily functioning, reduce daily pain, and manage pain flares that inevitably occur at work, after office hours, and on the weekends when a doctor visit is inconvenient. These techniques allow patients to gain a sense of self-control or self-efficacy over their pain, which is vital for long-term reduction in pain and disability *(13–15)*.

3.1. Physical Therapy

Most patients with chronic pain benefit from exercise that includes both a general aerobic conditioning program and targeted exercises for the specific pain syndrome. Exercise improves pain by enhancing general body conditioning, including improved structural support from muscles, joints, tendons, and ligaments, elevated endorphin levels, a general sense of well-being, weight reduction, and distraction from pain. Exercise programs are most effective if they are performed consistently, with aerobic exercise once a day and targeted stretches twice daily. Aerobic exercise may be performed outdoors, and stretching exercises may be completed while watching a daily television program. Combining exercise with a distracting and enjoyable activity improves long-term compliance. Patients must be careful when exercising with a partner that they choose someone whose exercise pace is similar to avoid over- or under-exercising.

Aerobic exercise may include walking, biking, or swimming. Walking programs are most convenient, and patients should be instructed in specific target goals. For example, patients may begin walking one-quarter of a mile daily for 4 to 5 days. Then their distance can be increased to one-half a mile daily or they might walk one-quarter of a mile twice daily. Walking distance can continue to be increased every 4 to 5 days until they are walking 1 to 2 miles daily. A faster or slower schedule may be used depending on baseline conditioning. Patients can easily identify distances by walking on high school tracks, in malls, or along routes they can measure with their car odometer. Table 6 shows a sample first week walking program (A), with completed logs for three patients (B). The first patient showed good compliance with the walking program, without a major increase in pain. Pain was mildly increased when the walking distance was first increased, but then returned to more moderate levels. The second patient underestimated his baseline conditioning, so he was advanced faster than originally planned, again without major pain flares. The third patient was noncompliant, missing walking days and trying to play "catch-up" by overdoing on some days. This resulted in major pain flares that caused the patient to spend a day in bed and then under-exercise on other days. This "crash-and-burn" pattern resulted in a referral to occupational therapy to learn pacing skills and better time management.

3.2. Occupational Therapy

Occupational therapy offers an evaluation of activities of daily living and work duties that may aggravate chronic pain complaints. After an activity assessment, the therapist can suggest ways to alter activities so that disability is maximized. For example, patients with low back pain aggravated by sitting at work may find that placing a brick under their feet when they sit improves posture and reduces pain. Similarly, a housewife whose pain is flared by vacuuming may be instructed to walk with the vacuum rather than pushing it out and pulling it back along the carpet. Simple devices, such as push carts for carrying supplies at work, may also be helpful.

Occupational therapists are also effective in teaching patients proper activity scheduling and pacing techniques to avoid over- or underdoing activities or a crash-and-burn pattern of too much activity with pain flares followed by severely restricted activities, as seen in the walking log for patient 3 in Table 6.

3.3. Psychological Treatment

Psychology for patients with chronic pain should focus on teaching pain management skills and addressing underlying psychological distress. The risk

Table 6
Sample Walking Logs

A. Schedule marked by ×s

	Sunday	Monday	Tuesday	Wednesday	Thursday	Friday	Saturday
1 mile							
¾ mile							
½ mile					×	×	×
¼ mile	×	×	×	×			

B. Completed logs

Patient 1[a]	Sunday	Monday	Tuesday	Wednesday	Thursday	Friday	Saturday
1 mile							
¾ mile							
½ mile					⊗ 6	⊗ 5	⊗ 4
¼ mile	⊗ 4	⊗ 5	⊗ 4	⊗ 4			

Patient 2[b]	Sunday	Monday	Tuesday	Wednesday	Thursday	Friday	Saturday
1 mile							
¾ mile						○ 6	○ 5
½ mile			○ 4	○ 5	⊗ 4	×	×
¼ mile	⊗ 3	⊗ 3	×	×			

Patient 3[c]	Sunday	Monday	Tuesday	Wednesday	Thursday	Friday	Saturday
1 mile							
¾ mile					○ 7		
½ mile					×	×	×
¼ mile	⊗ 4	×	⊗ 4	×			○ 5

[a] Patient 1: compliant with regimen, pacing acceptable.
[b] Patient 2: initial program underestimated exercise potential; program successfully accelerated.
[c] Patient 3: poor compliance with poor pacing and resultant pain flares.
Prescribed schedule is marked by ×s. Patients circle the actual distance walked and record their pain level from 0 (*no pain*) to 10 (*excruciating pain*) after walking next to the distance actually walked.

for depression or anxiety is four times greater in adults with chronic pain compared with pain-free controls *(16)*. If depression and anxiety are severe, psychiatric treatment may need to precede pain management because severe distress will impair the patient's ability to fully participate in effectively learning and implementing new skills.

Pain management techniques include the following:

- Relaxation training.
- Coping skills.
- Stress management.
- Cognitive restructuring.

Table 7
Effects of Cognitive Restructuring: Patient Experienced
a Severe Pain Flare After Driving Across the State for a Family Reunion

Thoughts before treatment	Thoughts after treatment
• I knew I should never have come. I should have just stayed home in bed. I'll never be able to visit my family again. • I'm sure I'll have this excruciating pain forever. • Why can't my doctor do anything to get my pain under control. It's just hopeless.	• Next time I drive 5 miles, I'd better plan to stop several times along the way to do some stretching exercises and walk a little. • When I get to my aunt's, I'll ask for some ice and do my stretching exercises. My pain may still be flared up in the morning, but it should be better by lunch time as long as I get up early for some relaxation, my stretches, and a walk.

Cognitive restructuring describes a change in thoughts from negative to positive. For example, most patients with chronic pain experience times where pain levels increase or flare, possibly related to an activity or for unknown reasons. Compare a patient's thoughts before and after treatment when experiencing a pain flare (Table 7). Notice the pretreatment paralyzing catastrophic thinking is adjusted to more appropriate thoughts after treatment that encourages the patient to use effective pain management skills.

Pain psychologists can also help patients adopt reasonable expectations from pain therapy. Unreasonable expectations include thinking that treatment should cure the pain or that medication alone is enough to keep pain under control. Even with effective pain management, most patients with chronic pain will continue to experience a mild-to-moderate level of pain every day, with occasional pain flares. Realistic goals include the following:

• Decreased daily pain to a more moderate level.
• Decreased frequency of pain flares.
• Decreased duration of pain flares.
• Increased level of activity/return to work.

For most patients, pain will occur whether they are at home or at work. Being at work improves their sense of well being, improves activity, and increases distractions from chronic pain. For these same reasons, children with chronic headache or other pains are encouraged to attend school regularly, even if they are having a headache or pain flare that day.

3.4. Healthy Lifestyle Recommendations

Following a healthy lifestyle improves both general health and chronic pain. Specific patient recommendations are provided in Box 1. Nicotine use, sleep disturbance, and obesity have been most directly linked to chronic pain occurrence and severity.

Box 1
Healthy Lifestyle Tips to Reduce Chronic Pain

1. Avoid nicotine

   Using cigarettes or other nicotine-containing products changes your body's levels of the natural pain-reliever endorphin. Smokers with a variety of chronic pain complaints, including migraine, myofascial pain, and other pain conditions, actually experience more frequent and severe pain than nonsmokers. Smoking did not cause you to get chronic pain. However, when you do have chronic pain, smoking makes the pain worse by interfering with your body's natural ability to reduce pain. Quitting smoking may reduce your pain after several weeks to months, when your body chemicals have readjusted.

   You may find it easier to quit smoking by using a nicotine patch, cutting down by one cigarette each week (if you smoke one pack daily, throw out one cigarette from each pack the first week, two cigarettes from each pack the second week, etc.), or quitting "cold turkey." The first step in designing an effective quitting strategy is to make sure you are sincerely committed to stopping smoking.

2. Sleep hygiene

   Sleep is often disrupted in people with chronic pain. Chronically poor sleep can worsen your mood, frustration, and pain tolerance. Some pain treatments, like antidepressants such as Elavil® (amitriptyline), also improve sleep. Steps to improve your sleep include the following:

   • Go to bed and rise at regular times.
   • Practice relaxation techniques before bed.
   • Do stretching exercises before bed.
   • Avoid caffeine after dinner.
   • Avoid watching television in bed.
   • Avoid napping or lying down during the day.

3. Weight management

   Increased weight puts added strain on muscles and joints. Interestingly, fat tissue also increases inflammation, which can further aggravate pain. Many people notice that losing even 5 to 15 pounds of extra weight can markedly improve their pain complaints. If you have a long-standing weight problem, losing weight and keeping it off can be hard. Strategies to improve your weight loss success include the following:

   • Do not skip meals. Schedule and eat six small meals throughout the day.
   • Reduce portion sizes and avoid taking seconds. If you are craving an extra helping after the meal, go for a walk or bike ride instead. If you cannot go outside, brush your teeth and do stretching exercises.
   • Limit television viewing to times when you are doing your stretching routine.
   • Schedule daily exercise. Find a walking partner so you can motivate each other and look forward to each other's company each day.
   • Eat breakfast cereal, nuts, hard boiled eggs, and fruit for snacks.

Box 1
Healthy Lifestyle Tips to Reduce Chronic Pain *(Continued)*

---

4. Aerobic exercise

Aerobic exercise improves muscle tone and joint flexibility. Aerobic exercise also increases endorphins, your body's natural pain killers. Increased endorphins makes aerobic instructors perky and helps marathon runners finish a grueling race. If you exercise daily, your endorphin levels will also increase, eventually causing pain to decrease.

Talk to your doctor before starting any exercise program to help determine what's best for you. Good aerobic exercise can include the following:

- Walking in the mall, on hiking trails, or on a school track.
- Biking.
- Swimming.

When you start any new aerobic program, begin slowly and increase the intensity about every 4 to 5 days. If your pain flares, temporarily reduce the activity to the level that you previously tolerated for about 2 to 3 days, then try increasing again.

Nicotine influences a variety of pain modulators, including endorphins *(17–19)* These data are supported by a recent study showing that smokers were more likely to use opioids than nonsmokers *(20)*. Therefore, it is not surprising that smokers are more likely to have a variety of chronic pain complaints than nonsmokers *(21)*. In one study, headache severity was linked to cigarette consumption, suggesting reducing nicotine use might decrease pain intensity *(22)*.

Sleep disturbance occurs in more than half of all patients with chronic pain *(23,24)*. Poor sleep has been consistently linked to depressed mood. Poor sleep also increases pain-related impairment, even after controlling for the effects of mood *(24,25)*. Sleep may be improved by using sleep hygiene techniques (Box 1) and some pain management medications (including antidepressants and anti-epileptics).

Obesity increases mechanical load on joints and increases proinflammatory cytokines that promote joint destruction *(28–28)* As expected, an increase in body weight increases the risk for developing osteoarthritis of the hand, hip, and knee *(29)*. Nonarthritic pain is also more prevalent in obese individuals. A large, longitudinal study of more than 6000 adults reported a significantly higher prevalence of musculoskeletal pain in obese versus nonobese adults (64% versus 35%) *(30)*. In addition, recovery from musculoskeletal pain after 2 years was significantly better in obese patients experiencing weight loss after bariatric surgery compared with those patients treated conventionally who did not experience significant weight loss. Several other studies have similarly demonstrated pain reduction after weight loss with surgical or nonsurgical treatments *(31–33)*.

4. SUMMARY

Improvements in chronic pain symptoms can be maximized by using a combination of medication and nonmedication techniques. Treatment should focus on reducing daily pain severity, pain flares, and disability. Allied heath care services can provide valuable self-management tools that allow patients with chronic pain to develop skills to gain control over their symptoms.

REFERENCES

1. McQuay HJ, Moore RA, Eccleston C, Morley S, de C Williams AC. Systematic review of outpatient services for chronic pain control. Health Technol Assess 1997;1:1–150.
2. Duman EN, Kesim M, Kadioglu M, et al. Possible involvement of opioidergic and serotonergic mechanisms in antinociceptive effect of paroxetine in acute pain. J Pharmacol Sci 2004;94:161–165.
3. Sindrup SH, Otto M, Finnerup NB, Jensen TS. Antidepressants in the treatment of neuropathic pain. Basic Clin Pharmacol Toxicl 2005;96:399–409.
4. Moja PL, Cusi C, Sterzi RR, Canepari C. Selective serotonin re-uptake inhibitors (SSRIs) for preventing migraine and tension-type headaches. Cochrane Database Syst Rev 2005;29:CD002919.
5. Reid MC, Engles-Horton LL, Weber MB, et al. Use of opioid medications for chronic noncancer pain syndromes in primary care. J Gen Intern Med 2002;17: 173–179.
6. Beers MH, Berkow R (Eds). Drug use and dependence. The Merck Manual of Diagnostics and Therapeutics, 17th Ed. Available at: www.merck.com/pubs. Accessed 11/13/05.
7. Lukaczer D, Darland G, Tripp M, et al. A pilot trial evaluating Meta050, a proprietary combination of reduced iso-alpha acids, rosemary extract and oleanic acid in patients with arthritis and fibromyalgia. Phytotherapy Res 2005;19:864–869.
8. Marcus DA. 10 Solutions to Migraine. Oakland, CA: New Harbinger Press, 2006.
9. Göbel H, Fresenius J, Heinze A, Dworschak M, Soyka D. Effectiveness of Oleum menthae piperitae and paracetamol in therapy of headache of the tension type. Nervenarzt 1996;67:672–681.
10. Peres MP, Zukerman E, da Cunha Tanuri F, Moreira FR, Cipolla-Neto J. Melatonin, 3 mg, is effective for migraine prevention. Neurology 2004;63:757.
11. Holroyd KA, Penzien DB. Pharmacological versus non-pharmacological prophylaxis of recurrent migraine headache: a meta-analytic review of clinical trials. Pain 1990;42:1–13.
12. Holroyd KA, O'Donnell FJ, Stensland M, et al. Management of chronic tension-type headache with tripcyclic antidepressant medication, stress management therapy, and their combination: a randomized controlled trial. JAMA 2001;285: 2208–2215.
13. Turner JA, Ersek M, Kemp C. Self–efficacy for managing pain is associated with disability, depression, and pain coping among retirement community residents with chronic pain. J Pain 2005;6:471–479.

14. Kool JP, Oesch PR, Bachman S, et al. Increasing days at work using function-centered rehabilitation in a nonacute nonspecific low back pain: a randomized controlled trial. Arch Phys Med Rehabil 2005;86:857–864.
15. McCahon S, Strong J, Sharry R, Cramond T. Self-report and pain behavior among patients with chronic pain. Clin J Pain 2005;21:223–231.
16. Gureje O, Von Korff M, Simon GE, Gater R. Persistent pain and well-being. A World Health Organization study in primary care. JAMA 1998;280:147–151.
17. Pomerleau OF. Endogenous opioids and smoking—a review of progress and problems. Psychoneuroendocrinolgy 1998;23:115–130.
18. Mansbach RS, Rovetti CC, Freeland CS. The role of monoamine neurotransmitters system in the nicotine discriminative stimulus. Drug Alcohol Depend 1998; 23:115–130.
19. Wewers ME, Dhatt RK, Snively TA, Tejwani GA. The effect of chronic administration of nicotine on antinociception, opioid receptor binding and met-enkephalin levels in rats. Brain Res 1999;822:107–113.
20. Rahimi-Movaghar V, Rakhshani F, Mohammadi M, Rahimi-Movaghar A. Opioid use in patients presenting with pain in Zahedan, Islamic Republic of Iran. East Mediterr Health J 2004;10:82–89.
21. Andersson H, Ejlertsson G, Leden I. Widespread musculoskeletal chronic pain associated with smoking. An epidemiological study in a general rural population. Scan J Rehabil Med 1998;30:185–191.
22. Payne TJ, Stetson B, Stevens VM, et al. Impact of cigarette smoking on headache activity in headache patients. Headache 1991;31:329–332.
23. Call-Schmidt TA, Richardson SJ. Prevalence of sleep disturbance and its relationship to pain in adults with chronic pain. Pain Manag Nurs 2003;4:124–133.
24. Morin CM, Gibson D, Wade J. Self-reported sleep and mood disturbance in chronic pain atients. Clin J Pain 1998;14:311–314.
25. Wilson KG, Eriksson MY, D'Eon JL, et al. Major depression and insomnia in chronic pain. Clin J Pain 2002;18:77–83.
26. Sharma L, Lou C, Cahue S, Dunlop DD. The mechanism of the effect of obesity in knee osteoarthritis: the mediating role of malalignment. Arthritis Rheum 2000; 43:568–75.
27. Bastard JP, Jardel C, Bruckett E, et al. Elevated levels of interleukin 6 are reduced in serum and subcutaneous adipose tissue of obese women after weight loss. J Clin Endocrinol Metab 2000;85:3338–3342.
28. Winkler G, Salamon F, Harmos G, et al. Elevated serum tumor necrosis factor-alpha concentrations and bioactivity in Type 2 diabetes and patients with android type obesity. Diabetes Res Clin Pract 1998;42:169–174.
29. Oliveria SA, Felson DT, Cirillo PA, Reed JI, Walker AM. Body weight, body mass index, and incident symptomatic osteoarthritis of the hand, hip, and knee. Epidemiology 1999;10:161–166.
30. Peltonen M, Lindroos AK, Torgerson JS. Musculoskeletal pain in the obese: a comparison with a general population and long-term changes after conventional and surgical obesity treatment. Pain 2003;104:549–557.
31. Evers Larsson U. Influence of weight loss on pain, perceived disability and observed functional limitations in obese women. Int J Obes Relat Metab Disord 2004;28:269–277.

32. Huang M, Chen C, Chen T, Weng M, Wang W, Wang Y. The effects of weight reduction on the rehabilitation of patients with knee osteoarthritis and obesity. Arthritis Care Res 2000;13:398–405.
33. Melissas J, Volakakis E, Hadjipavlou A. Low-back pain in morbidly obese patients and the effect of weight loss following surgery. Obes Surg 2003;13:389–393.

Index